W9-DBU-258

The Health Fitness Handbook

B. Don Franks, PhD
Edward T. Howley, PhD
Yuruk Iyriboz, MD

WITHDRAWN FROM LIBRARY

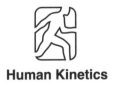

Human Kinetics

255791

MAR 2 8 2001

Library of Congress Cataloging-in-Publication Data

Franks, B. Don.
 The health fitness handbook / B. Don Franks, Edward T. Howley, and
Yuruk Iyriboz.
  p. cm.
 Includes bibliographical references and index.
 ISBN 0-88011-651-X
  1. Physical fitness--Handbooks, manuals, etc.   2. Exercise-
-Handbooks, manuals, etc.   3. Health--Handbooks, manuals, etc.
I. Howley, Edward T., 1943-   . II. Iyriboz, Yuruk, 1937-   .
III. Title.
RA781.F675 1999
613.7--dc21   98-52988
                                                                        CIP

ISBN: 0-88011-651-X

Copyright © 1999 by B. Don Franks, Edward T. Howley, and Yuruk Iyriboz

All rights reserved. Except for use in a review, the reproduction or utilization of this work in any form or by any electronic, mechanical, or other means, now known or hereafter invented, including xerography, photocopying, and recording, and in any information storage and retrieval system, is forbidden without the written permission of the publisher.

Notice: Permission to reproduce the following material is granted to instructors and agencies who have purchased *The Health Fitness Handbook*: tables 1, 2, 10.2, 10.3, 10.4, and 10.5. The reproduction of other parts of this book is expressly forbidden by the above copyright notice. Persons or agencies who have not purchased *The Health Fitness Handbook* may not reproduce any material.

Acquisitions Editor: Martin Barnard; **Managing Editor:** Coree Schutter; **Assistant Editor:** Laurie Stokoe; **Copyeditor:** Patricia Fortney; **Proofreader:** Myla Smith; **Indexer:** Theresa Schaefer; **Graphic Designer:** Robert Reuther; **Graphic Artist:** Francine Hamerski; **Photo Editor:** Amy Outland; **Cover Designer:** Jack Davis; **Photographer (interior):** Tom Roberts, unless otherwise indicated; **Illustrator:** Tom Roberts; **Printer:** Versa Press

Human Kinetics books are available at special discounts for bulk purchase. Special editions or book excerpts can also be created to specification. For details, contact the Special Sales Manager at Human Kinetics.

Printed in the United States of America   10 9 8 7 6 5 4 3 2 1

Human Kinetics
Web site: http://www.humankinetics.com/

United States: Human Kinetics
P.O. Box 5076, Champaign, IL 61825-5076
1-800-747-4457
e-mail: humank@hkusa.com

Canada: Human Kinetics
475 Devonshire Road Unit 100
Windsor, ON N8Y 2L5
1-800-465-7301 (in Canada only)
e-mail: humank@hkcanada.com

Europe: Human Kinetics
P.O. Box IW14, Leeds LS16 6TR
United Kingdom
+44 (0)113-278 1708
e-mail: humank@hkeurope.com

Australia: Human Kinetics
57A Price Avenue, Lower Mitcham
South Australia 5062
(08) 82771555
e-mail: humank@hkaustralia.com

New Zealand: Human Kinetics
P.O. Box 105-231, Auckland Central
09-523-3462
e-mail: humank@hknewz.com

To our children and grandchildren

Alice Evelyn Franks
Ray Martin Franks
Elizabeth Franks-North
Emily Franks-North

Sean Howley
Chris Howley
Geoffrey Howley
Luke Howley
Kayla Howley

Elif Iyriboz
Ayse Iyriboz

Contents

Preface

Is it dangerous to jog?
I can't get fit because I'm not good at sports.
What and how much fluid should I drink after exercise?
I've been exercising for weeks and haven't lost a pound!
Would it be better to do weight training every day?
If I'm feeling poorly, should I go ahead with my workout?

These are some of the comments and questions we have heard over the years while working with individuals in fitness programs and medical clinics. Noticing a growing interest in looking good, losing weight, and being fit—all in safe and healthy ways—we developed *The Health Fitness Handbook* (the second edition of *Fitness Facts*) to help answer the questions and address the frustrations voiced to us by potential fitness participants. This book provides information directly to individuals as they attempt to increase health and fitness, whether on their own or as part of a fitness program. If an individual is interested in a fitness program, this book can be used along with companion books written for fitness professionals (*Health Fitness Instructor's Handbook*, now in its third edition) and exercise leaders (*Fitness Leader's Handbook*, now in its second edition).

Since the publication of the first edition, numerous official statements and reports have supported the importance of regular physical activity, including *Healthy People 2000 Goals*, published by the U.S. Department of Health and Human Services; *NIH Consensus Development Conference on Physical Activity and Cardiovascular Health*; a position statement on the importance of physical activity by the Center for Disease Control and Prevention, the American College of Sports Medicine, and the President's Council on Physical Fitness and Sports; and an extensive review of current research evidence on *Physical Activity and Health* from the office of the U.S. Surgeon General. In addition, groups such as the American Heart Association and the American Medical Association have recognized that physical inactivity is a major risk factor for cardiovascular and other health problems.

In developing *The Health Fitness Handbook,* we used these position statements and research reviews to update our recommendations for safe and effective physical activity for those interested in promoting their own health and fitness. Although it is written in simple, straightforward, and understandable language, the concepts are based on the latest research and professional opinion.

The Health Fitness Handbook describes the components of fitness related to health. It teaches you how to evaluate and improve your current health and fitness status, giving helpful hints on preventing injury and changing other health-related behaviors. Practical tips have been inserted throughout the book to give you additional information about becoming fit safely.

Two of the authors, Don Franks and Ed Howley, have PhD degrees with three decades of experience in research, teaching, and working directly with fitness tests and activities. They are joined by Yuruk Iyriboz for the second edition. Dr. Iyriboz is an MD with a master of public health degree from Johns Hopkins University. He has practiced medicine for more than 34 years and currently is director of an urgi-care clinic that emphasizes helping patients prevent major health problems through good nutrition, physical activity, and the use of medication only as needed. All three authors have been active in professional organizations and in efforts to enhance the health and fitness of all people.

The authors benefit from an active lifestyle. We wrote *The Health Fitness Handbook* to share the fun, the advantages, and the necessary precautions of physical activity. If, as a result of reading this book, some individuals experience an enhanced quality of life by participating safely in enjoyable activities, our time was well spent.

Acknowledgments

Thanks to David Bassett, Jr., Vernon Bond, Jr., Janet Buckworth, Sue Carver, Jean Lewis, Wendell Liemohn, Daniel Martin, and Dixie Thompson. Their contributions to the third edition of the *Health Fitness Instructor's Handbook* were invaluable to us as we developed this book.

We would also like to thank the many fitness professionals who have provided helpful suggestions for this revised edition, in addition to the authors and publishers who were kind enough to allow us to use materials from their articles and books. We are indebted to our former professors; our students; and professional colleagues in AAHPERD, ACSM, and AAKPE, too numerous to list, who have educated us over the past three decades.

Finally, thanks to the folks at Human Kinetics: Rainer Martens, Julie Martens, Martin Barnard, and Coree Schutter, who have provided encouragement and assistance in many ways.

Introduction

We all deal with our fitness and health on some level. The question is, do we approach them directly and intelligently, are we persuaded by the best advertising, or do we simply let our fitness and health be determined by default from decisions in other areas of our lives?

In the following pages we provide a number of tables to assist in your fitness assessment. We strongly encourage you to complete these tables honestly and as completely as possible. You can submit these tables to the fitness leader if you are in a fitness program, or you can use the information for self-evaluation.

Determining your level of satisfaction with your current health and fitness status will provide a start for deciding what areas of your life you want to change. This book provides the information you need to set up your own fitness program. Or you may decide to work with health and fitness professionals to assist you in making healthy changes in your life. In either case, you have to decide what you want to change. The old joke, "How many psychologists does it take to change a light bulb? Only one, but it has to really want to change!" applies to fitness changes as well.

Complete table 1 to identify your degree of satisfaction with different aspects of fitness and your life (e.g., your amount of energy, cardiovascular endurance, amount of body fat, strength, ability to relax, ability to sleep, blood pressure, physical appearance). These items should point out areas of your life you want to change (see table 2) and help you (or the fitness leader) establish special emphases in your fitness program. Looking at how your answers to these questions have changed three months or a year from now can help you evaluate and modify your fitness activities.

Table 1

Degree of Satisfaction With Different Aspects of Fitness

Circle the best number for each aspect of your fitness level, using this scale:

4 = Very satisfied
3 = Satisfied
2 = Dissatisfied
1 = Very dissatisfied

Amount of energy	4	3	2	1
Cardiovascular endurance	4	3	2	1
Blood pressure	4	3	2	1
Amount of body fat	4	3	2	1
Strength	4	3	2	1
Ability to cope with tension/stress	4	3	2	1
Ability to relax	4	3	2	1
Ability to sleep	4	3	2	1
Posture	4	3	2	1
Low back function	4	3	2	1
Physical appearance	4	3	2	1
Overall physical fitness	4	3	2	1
Level of regular medication	4	3	2	1

Note: From *The Health Fitness Handbook* by B.D. Franks and E.T. Howley, 1999, Champaign, IL: Human Kinetics. This form may be copied by instructors and agencies who have purchased this book.

Table 2

Things That Bother Me

List the things that you want to change:

Specific physical problem:

Appearance of particular part of body:

Ability to play a specific sport:

Risk of a health problem:

Other:

Note: From *The Health Fitness Handbook* by B.D. Franks and E.T. Howley, 1999, Champaign, IL: Human Kinetics. This form may be copied by instructors and agencies who have purchased this book.

Can This Book Help?

The answer depends on the behavior(s) you want to change. Read the rest of this introduction to discover if the things you are not happy about and plan to change in your life are components of physical fitness. If they are, we can help you.

Total Fitness

The term *fitness* has been applied to many different goals—the avoidance of disease, efficiency in everyday life, the ability to do certain activities at desired levels (e.g., dance, sports), and healthy mental and social behaviors. Total fitness is the capacity to combine all of these aspects to achieve the optimal quality of life. The fully fit person has high levels of cardiorespiratory function and mental alertness; meaningful social relationships; the ability to cope with problems; desirable levels of fat; sufficient levels of flexibility, muscular strength, and endurance; and a healthy low back. If you are fit, your life includes regular exercise and a healthy diet, and you are able to cope with stressors without substance abuse. Being fit means being able to enjoy a full life with a low risk of developing major health problems.

People can achieve fitness goals up to their *genetic potential*—an individual's inherited capacity for both health and performance. It is impossible, however, to determine exactly how much of your health or performance is determined by heredity and how much by development. Most people can lead healthy or unhealthy lives regardless of their inheritance. Thus your particular genetic background neither dooms you to low fitness levels nor guarantees high fitness levels.

Certain aspects of our *environment* can be controlled: many of the mental and physical exercises we do are a matter of choice. But we are all limited in certain ways by our past and current environments. For example, some people are hungry as a result of their environments and obviously can't think about other aspects of fitness until basic food needs are fulfilled. The degree to which fitness can be changed depends in part on when a person starts. For example, children who are active and eat well develop fewer fat cells than children who lead sedentary lives and have poor eating habits. Most adults are stuck with the number of fat cells they developed as children and, later in life, can only change the size of those cells.

Total fitness is *dynamic*; it involves striving, growing, developing, and becoming. It can never be "achieved" in the fullest sense; the fit person is continually approaching the highest quality of life possible. This book focuses on the *physical fitness* aspects of positive health. However, it is appropriate to discuss briefly the broader picture, so that our physical fitness emphasis can be put into perspective regarding other aspects of fitness, health, and performance.

Fitness, Health, and Performance

The four layers of physical fitness, health, and performance—lack of disease, everyday efficiency, physical fitness, and performance—build on one another. Freedom from disease and the ability to get through one's daily routine can provide the base for starting a fitness program to achieve a higher level of positive health and reduce the risk of health problems. Those interested in performing at high levels in sports or developing other physical skills can build on the fitness base by concentrating on ways to improve their performance.

Health Risks

Mental, emotional, and physical health serve as a base for everyone's total fitness. Regular exercise, a healthy diet, living without substance abuse, and coping with stressors can reduce many of the primary and secondary risks to health. In addition to helping prevent health problems, these behaviors are the basis for a higher quality of life.

In order to become fit we must understand the characteristics and behaviors related to positive and negative health. *Primary* risk factors, such as smoking, high concentrations of serum low-density lipoprotein cholesterol (LDL-C), low concentrations of serum high-density lipoprotein cholesterol (HDL-C), high blood pressure, physical inactivity, and diabetes, are strongly associated with a particular health problem independent of all other variables. On the other hand, *secondary* risk factors, such as obesity, a high-fat diet, an inability to cope with stress, a coronary-prone personality, and high triglyceride levels, contribute to the health problem only when other factors are present. Risk factors can also be classified as those that are inherited and unalterable and those that result from lifestyle behaviors and can be modified.

What Risks Are Unavoidable?

Some risk factors are easily identified but unfortunately can't be altered. For example, certain segments of the population—those with a family history of the disease, older people, and men—have a greater risk of heart disease, especially if they adopt unhealthy behaviors. It is important to point out that these are secondary risk factors for heart disease, resulting in a high risk only when added to other risk factors.

The risk associated with family history and age can be lessened by behavior changes. Family history often includes unhealthy dietary, activity, smoking, and stress behaviors that tend to be transmitted from parents to children. In terms of aging, research has shown that many fitness characteristics (e.g., cardiovascular function, percent body fat) deteriorate with each passing decade. This decline, which starts in the middle 20s, has been called the "aging curve." However, the decline in cardiorespiratory function and the increase in body fat occurs partly because older individuals lead less active lives—not because of aging itself. By maintaining an active lifestyle we can slow down the fitness decline seen in typical aging curves.

Healthy Low Back

A healthy low back is an important component of fitness. Many fitness activities are impossible to pursue if back problems are present. Clinical evidence points to several risk factors associated with the development of low back problems: lack of abdominal muscle endurance, lack of flexibility in the midtrunk region and the back of the thighs, poor posture (lying, sitting, standing, moving), poor lifting habits, and an inability to cope with stress.

Health and Fitness Goals

Research shows that we can enhance our health by participating in regular physical activity; eating a well-rounded and nutritious diet; maintaining recommended levels of body fat (through exercise and diet); learning to cope with stressors; and enjoying life without smoking, excess alcohol, or other drugs.

Fitness also includes dealing with the unique aspects of our individual lives. Some of us must maintain certain body positions and postures for extended periods of time either at home or at work, while others must perform various levels and types of physical activity. Our leisure activities may make different physical demands. Thus our plans for a healthier life should include not only the healthy behaviors essential for everyone but also specific activities designed to benefit our regular activities at work, at home, and at play.

Gaining Control of Health

While the promise of improving your health and becoming fit can be exciting, changing unhealthy lifestyles can be difficult and frustrating. Starting a fitness program, however, puts you at the cutting edge of health and can help you gain control of your life. Such control begins with an evaluation of risk factors and behaviors related to health, which you will find in chapter 1.

The Exercise and Health Checklist

In order to attain fitness you must first be fully aware of your current health status. Starting a fitness program without this awareness is in itself a risk. You should be aware of the following:

- Known medical problems
- Characteristics that increase the risk of health problems
- Signs or symptoms indicative of health problems
- Lifestyle behaviors related to health problems
- Any problems that interfere with activities of daily life
- Results of a physical fitness evaluation

Because we tend to forget our medical problems until we have serious conditions that require daily medications and frequent visits to a physician, it is best to keep a copy of all medical records. They can be obtained easily from your physician. Your parents can also be very helpful in providing information on your medical history. Even if you are in excellent shape, your medical history is very important since injuries that occur during exercise may require immediate medical attention. You need to know the date of your last immunizations, especially your tetanus shot, as well as any allergic reactions to medicine.

Evaluation of Health Status

You should now complete the Health Status Questionnaire found in Appendix A on pages 179–182. The following sections will help you focus on different aspects of your health and fitness status as reflected in the questionnaire.

Health Problems

Questions 12 to 15 should remind you of any known health problems that may affect your exercise program. If you checked any of the items in questions 12 to 15, you will need to work closely with the fitness instructor and your physician to ensure that you are involved in physical activities that are healthy for you. If you are on certain medications, changing your exercise habits may require close monitoring of medication levels and your diet as you work with your physician and fitness instructor.

Characteristics That Are Health-Related Risks

As we mentioned earlier, you have a higher risk of cardiovascular disease or stroke if your relatives (especially parents, question 10) had cardiovascular disease or stroke prior to age 55. You also have a higher risk if you are male. All of us have increased risk of major health problems as we grow older. Any of these characteristics should make you more determined to adopt healthy behaviors and change unhealthy practices.

Health-Related Signs/Symptoms

Question 15 on the Health Status Questionnaire includes some of the signs and symptoms that could indicate a major health problem. If you have any of these signs or symptoms, do not begin a fitness program until you have discussed them with your physician to determine if they reflect a problem that needs medical attention.

Healthy and Unhealthy Behaviors

Questions 16 to 23 are related to healthy and unhealthy behaviors. Your habits related to exercise, eating, smoking, the use of alcohol and other drugs, and your ability to cope with stress are important elements in your health status.

Fitness Test Results and Health

If you are involved in a good fitness program, you will be taking a number of physical fitness tests as you go along. It is not important for you to perform better than everyone else on these tests, but it is important for you to be in the optimal range for percent body fat, have adequate levels of cardiorespiratory function, and develop sufficient abdominal strength/endurance and midtrunk flexibility to minimize the risk of low back problems.

Ask your fitness leader to explain how your test results relate to health standards. If you are on a do-it-yourself fitness program, you can chart your progress in various ways. Can you walk, jog, or cycle at a moderate pace for longer periods without fatigue? Do everyday tasks such as climbing stairs, taking out the trash, or reaching for an object seem easier? If you had excess fat and have been doing fitness activities for several weeks, do you notice a difference in the way your clothes fit? Do you recover from physical exertion more easily? Do

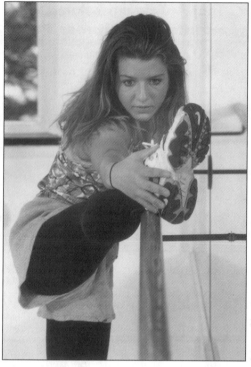

© Terry Wild Studio

you have more energy late in the day? Are you sleeping better? Do you feel better than you did before you started your exercise program? A good fitness program results in your answering "yes" to many of these questions and will also teach you important lifestyle changes such as healthy eating, good posture, and proper lifting techniques.

Now that you have evaluated your current health status, it is time to consider the next steps in starting your fitness program.

Starting Your Fitness Program

When most folks decide that they want to begin a fitness program, they think immediately of what activities they will do. Participation in fitness activities, however, should be preceded by other important steps. The different aspects of a fitness program are listed in table 1.1.

Table 1.1

Components of a Fitness Program

Sequence of decisions for fitness

1. Deciding to do something
2. Determining health status
3. Seeking professional advice
4. Selecting a fitness program
5. Undergoing additional screening
6. Undergoing fitness testing
7. Participating in fitness activities
8. Undergoing periodic testing
9. Modifying fitness activities

Moving From Health Status Evaluation to a Fitness Program

People that have been diagnosed with and are being treated for major health problems can work with their physicians to determine appropriate fitness programs. Those who have carefully analyzed their health status and know that they have no health problems or unhealthy behaviors can create a fitness program based on their interests. Many of us, however, fall between these two extremes—we may not have a major health problem, but we probably have a variety of risk factors that affect our health status.

Before beginning a fitness program, you need to decide, perhaps with the assistance of a fitness professional, whether you should get medical clearance. The *current standard* suggests that people with known health problems or signs or symptoms indicative of potential health problems consult a physician prior to beginning a fitness program. In addition, older people and anyone planning to engage in very strenuous athletic activities (in which the intensity is much higher than that needed for fitness gains) should have medical clearance prior to participation. The next few sections will help you proceed from thinking about your health status to making a decision about your next step.

Should I Check With a Physician?

If you have been told that you have a major cardiovascular or other health problem that would interfere with regular exercise or if you are taking medications for high blood pressure or some other health problem (such as diabetes or asthma) that might affect your exercise, you should consult your physician about any limitations to your exercise. Your physician may know of a supervised exercise program for people with your health problem. Table 1.2 will help you determine whether to seek medical advice prior to beginning a fitness program, enroll in a supervised program, include special precautions while exercising, or set up your own program.

If there is any question in your mind, ask your physician first. Based on her or his recommendation, you can make one of the following decisions:

1. Obtain immediate medical attention for a health problem prior to starting a fitness program.
2. Enroll in a fitness program that is
   - medically supervised,
   - carefully prescribed and supervised by a fitness instructor or offered by a fitness center, or
   - done individually.

A good fitness program begins with a battery of tests to determine your cardiorespiratory function and body composition. If your values are outside the range of those listed in table 1.2, then medical referral is recommended. Chapters 5 through 7 include detailed recommendations for fitness testing.

Fitness Program Guidelines

The values listed as bases for medical referral and supervised programs are guidelines to be used along with other information supplied by you and the fitness program director. Since some variables may be influenced by your pretest activities and your reaction to the testing situation itself (some people are not comfortable in the testing environment), borderline scores, especially at rest and during light activity,

Table 1.2

Conditions and Test Score Criteria for Physical Activity Decisions

BASIS FOR MEDICAL REFERRAL

Conditions

Shortness of breath with slight exertion	Head trauma
Cirrhosis	Heart, brain, or abdomen operation, disease, or problem
Coughing up blood	Pain in the abdomen, joint, extremities, or chest
Current medication for heart, blood pressure, diabetes, or asthma	Phlebitis
Faintness or dizziness	Stroke

Test Scores[a]

Resting HR > 90 bpm	Cholesterol/HDL > 5
Resting SBP > 160 mmHg	Triglycerides > 200 mg/dl
Resting DBP > 100 mmHg	Fasting glucose > 120 mg/dl
% fat > 40 female; > 30 male	Vital capacity < 75% predicted
Cholesterol > 240 mg/dl	Forced expiratory volume in one second < 75%

BASIS FOR A SUPERVISED PROGRAM

Conditions (currently under control)[b]

Alcoholism	Drug abuse	Low back pain
Allergy	Emphysema	Mental illness
Anemia	Epilepsy	Mononucleosis
Asthma	Fibromyalgia	Peptic ulcer
Bleeding trait	Fractures/sprains	Post-traumatic stress disorder
Bronchitis	Head trauma	
Cancer	Hepatitis/kidney disease	Pregnancy
Colitis	Hypoglycemia	Thyroid problem
Diabetes	Ligament/tendon tears	

Test Scores[c]

Hypertension (BP) 140–159/90–99 mmHg	Waist-to-hip ratio > 0.8 female; > 0.9 male
Hyperlipidemia (cholesterol) 240–255 mg/dl	Smoking > 20 cigarettes/day
Cholesterol/HDL 4.5–4.8	Exercise < 1.5 hr/week at or above moderate intensity
Obesity (% fat) 32–38% female; 25–28% male	

(continued)

Table 1.2   (continued)

BASIS FOR SPECIAL ATTENTION

Conditions

Allergies	Inability to maintain certain postures
Arthritis	Inability to perform certain motions
Back, eye, joint, lung, or neck operations	Lengthy time spent driving, lifting, sitting, or standing
Eye problems	
Hearing loss	Low back pain
Hernia	Repetitive motions
Stress due to cold, humidity, or heat	Sensitivity to dust or sunlight

Test Scores

Values of risk factors approaching those in supervised programs

Any of the reasons for stopping a maximal test that occur at light to moderate work

Max RPE < 5 (or < 15 on 6–20 scale)

Max METs < 8

Max $\dot{V}O_2$ < 30

% fat < 15% or > 30% females; < 6% or > 25% males[d]

Curl-ups < 10

Sit-and-reach < 15 cm

Modified pull-ups < 5

Push-ups < 10

Note. Any condition or test value that causes the person or the HFI to be concerned for the person's health or safety is the basis for medical referral.

FEV_1 = forced expiratory volume in 1 s; RPE = rating of perceived exertion.

[a] Any of these individual scores would be the basis for referral. A person might also be referred if more than one test score approached these values.

[b] Severe or uncontrolled levels should be referred for medical attention.

[c] Persons with higher scores should be referred for medical attention.

[d] Participants who have either too little fat or too much fat may have health problems that need special attention. If there is any question, refer them to the program director.

Reprinted, by permission, from E.T. Howley and B.D. Franks, 1997, *Health Fitness Instructor's Handbook*, 3d ed. (Champaign, IL: Human Kinetics), 40–41.

should be replicated before medical referral. For example, if you had a high resting heart rate or high resting blood pressure, it may have been because you ate, smoked, took medicine, or participated in physical exercise just prior to the test. Were you anxious about taking the test? Were there unusual conditions during the test (lots of people, noise, etc.)? The fitness instructor may have you rest for a few minutes, reassure you about the purpose and safety of the test, and test you again, or you may be rescheduled for another day. If the questionable test result is repeated, then you may be referred to a health care specialist.

It is important to note that the categories listed in table 1.2 are not hard and fast. A person categorized as needing a supervised program may actually need to be medically referred if, for example, he or she has multiple risk factors, each close to the referral value. Or the medical consultant may recommend that someone in our "refer" category enter a supervised program, based on a recent medical examination or conversation with a personal physician. Programs with excellent and accessible medical and emergency personnel may use higher values for referral than do programs isolated from medical and emergency facilities.

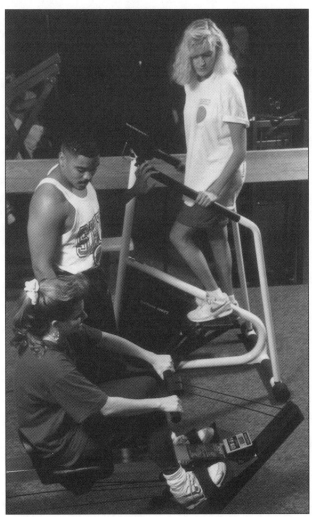

© Terry Wild Studio

Supervised Programs

Table 1.2 also lists mild or moderate levels of the conditions and test scores that would suggest you can participate in a carefully supervised fitness program, and identifies characteristics that call for special attention or limited activities. It is important that the exercise leader be informed of these or other conditions that may be related to your ability to exercise.

Self-Initiated Fitness Activities

If you are free of the health problems, conditions, or behaviors we've listed that require medical referral or supervised programs; have no questionable responses to fitness tests; and have no other reason to question your ability to begin a fitness program, then you can participate in any of the fitness activities in this book (using the recommended levels of work) with minimal risk. Your major goals will be to improve or maintain your fitness level through activities that provide an appropriate fitness stimulus and are enjoyable to you. You may want to try some new activities to add variety to your workouts.

Now that you have evaluated your health status and considered your risk factors or lack thereof, you can use this information to increase healthy behaviors, including a safe and appropriate fitness program.

chapter 2

Changing Old Behaviors

Are you physically active for 30 minutes every day? Do you exercise at least three times a week at a moderate to vigorous intensity for 30 to 40 minutes each workout? Do you smoke? Do you have more than a couple of drinks a week? Do you take other drugs or medicine on a regular basis? Is your weight what it should be? Do you eat a well-balanced diet? Are you able to cope with day-to-day stress? Can you deal with big emotional problems when they arise? Do you rely on eating, drinking, and/or drugs when problems arise? If your answers to these questions reflect a healthy lifestyle, then you can skip this chapter. Most of us, however, have one or more habits that prevent us from achieving our highest possible levels of fitness and health. In fact, as a society we could make great strides in public health if we changed several aspects of the typical U.S. lifestyle.

If you have thought about changing the way you live so you can be healthier, then this chapter can help you. The chapter focuses on five behaviors that are directly related to health: smoking, alcohol intake, weight, stress, and exercise. The first part of the chapter addresses behavior modification. The rest of the chapter discusses the causes of specific unhealthy behaviors and ways to deal with them.

Stages of Change

One popular way to understand how to change behavior (called the Transtheoretical Model of Behavior Change) lists five stages:

1. Precontemplation
2. Contemplation
3. Preparation
4. Action
5. Maintenance

Determining which stage applies to each of your health-related behaviors can be helpful. If you are not thinking seriously about making a change in the next few months (*precontemplation*), then you need to read or talk with a professional in that area to determine if a need exists for you to change. If you are considering making a change soon (*contemplation*), then you should explore the possibilities of how such a change might be accomplished in your life.

For those areas in which you have decided to make a change immediately (*preparation*), you need to identify your current status, set some long- and short-term goals, and get professional help (if needed) to determine the dimensions of your new behavior. For example, what type, how much, how frequently, and for how long are you going to engage in physical activity tomorrow? What specific changes are you going to make in your usual breakfast, lunch, dinner, and snacks tomorrow? You may want to sign a contract with a friend indicating your specific intentions.

In the *action* stage, you have begun your new activity. You need to monitor your new behavior; get help from friends to continue your behavior; and plan how you can continue the behavior tomorrow and in the next few days, weeks, and months.

For healthy behaviors that are now a part of your lifestyle, you need to plan ways to continue them (*maintenance*). This involves continuing to monitor the behavior, periodically reassessing what you are doing to determine whether adjustments are needed, and anticipating situations in which it will be difficult to continue the behavior (e.g., if you have stopped drinking for almost a year and will be attending a New Year's Eve party next week). Figure 2.1 offers intervention strategies for the various stages of change.

Changing Behavior

Later in the chapter, we discuss the problems of inactivity, smoking, alcoholism, excess fat, and stress and recommend some specific procedures for resolving them. Before doing that, though, we will present a general plan with a variety of steps you can take to help you adopt

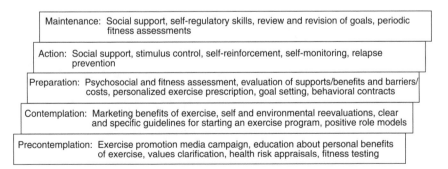

Figure 2.1 Intervention strategies for various areas of change.
Reprinted, by permission, from E.T. Howley and B.D. Franks, *Health Fitness Instructor's Handbook*, 3d ed. (Champaign, IL: Human Kinetics), 392.

healthy behaviors. This general plan has several components, but you won't necessarily use each step for every habit you want to change. A procedure that helps you to resolve one particular problem may not work for someone else, and it may not help you resolve other problems. The steps outlined in table 2.1 provide a general plan of steps that can be reduced, added to, or modified depending on what works for you. The general plan is also a preview of the procedures to modify specific behaviors that we discuss in later portions of this chapter.

As you begin to make changes in your life, don't feel that you have to do it alone—ask for help. Choose someone who is a good role model for the desired behavior and who will be supportive of you as you make changes.

Your fitness instructor, a counselor, or a close friend are good choices for people to enlist to help you throughout the process. The first step is to *analyze the problem.* Analysis includes facing such questions as when the behavior started, what the conditions were when it started, why it continues, when it last happened, and under what conditions. If you have had difficulty changing a certain behavior in the past, you

Table 2.1

General Model for Changing Behavior

Step	Activity
1	Acknowledge desire to change.
2	Analyze history of problem.
3	Record current behavior.
4	Analyze current status.
5	Set long-term goals.
6	Set short-term goals.
7	Sign contract with friend(s).
8	List many possible strategies that could be used.
9	Select one or two strategies to use.
10	Learn new coping skills.
11	Establish regular contact with helper.
12	Once goal is reached, outline potential maintenance problems.
13	Learn new coping skills.
14	Maintain periodic contact with helper.

Reprinted, by permission, from E.T. Howley and B.D. Franks, 1986, *Health Fitness Instructor's Handbook* (Champaign, IL: Human Kinetics), 200.

may feel fearful and helpless about trying to change again. Express these feelings to your helper and ask for help in going forward in spite of these feelings. Both you and your helper need to reach a mutual understanding of the problem. Collecting some baseline data concerning the extent of the behavior over a period of several days often aids this analysis. After the initial analysis, you should be able to describe clearly the current status of the problem.

Once you have analyzed the past and present, address the future by discussing your *goals*. Goal statements concern future conditions and often include time constraints. You suggest your desired goal, and your helper assists in making the goal realistic and clear. If you are making a major behavior change, subgoals are advisable. Achieving the goal of successful behavior for a single day may lead to two successful days, then three, a week, and so on. For example, your long-term goal may be to walk for 30 minutes at least five days per week. Your subgoal might be to take two 10-minute exercise breaks Monday through Friday next week. To increase the chances of achieving the goal, you can offer yourself a reward when the goal is achieved.

Signing a contract has also helped individuals achieve their goals. A written agreement, specifying the conditions to be met and the rewards or consequences if it is or is not met, is more successful if it is made between the individual who wants to change and a close friend. Some contracts are for taking positive steps (e.g., beginning exercise). Other contracts are for avoiding negative behavior (e.g., smoking). In some cases, contracts are made among a group of individuals who support each other and increase everyone's level of commitment.

Once you have analyzed a problem and agreed to a goal, the next step is to determine a *plan* for reaching the goal. The first step in developing a plan is for you and your helper to brainstorm—list as many different plans as possible without taking time to evaluate each one. From this list, pick the one or two *strategies* that seem to have the best chance of success. Depending on the strategy you select, you may need to learn new coping behaviors, such as how to relax or how to be more assertive.

After you have reached an initial goal, a very difficult stage is entered: namely, *maintaining* long-term results. Recognizing the environmental conditions under which old behaviors are likely to occur increases your chances of taking steps to avoid them. Long-term contact between you and your helper can maintain the change over time. This contact can become less frequent as your new behavior(s) becomes part of your lifestyle.

Starting and Maintaining Physical Activity

The 1990, 2000, and projected 2010 health objectives for the United States include a threefold increase in appropriate aerobic exercise in the adult population. Exercise seems to benefit us both physiologically and psychologically. Chapter 10 deals with specific factors (e.g., intensity) needed for improvement in health-related fitness as well as a variety of activities that can be used for fitness.

The current emphasis on and interest in fitness has brought many people (like you) into fitness programs. A major problem for many is sticking with it; in many programs up to 50 percent of participants quit within six months. People more likely to drop out include those who smoke, have low self-motivation, lack social reinforcement, and believe that additional exercise is unnecessary. The reasons often given for quitting exercise are inconvenience and lack of time. One method to help you increase and maintain your adherence to exercise is to join an exercise program with the following characteristics:

1. *Availability.* Change is facilitated by accessible programs. Find a program with convenient times and a convenient location.

2. *Social support.* When you include your family and/or "significant others" (i.e., persons important to you such as your spouse,

BENEFITS OF PHYSICAL ACTIVITY

Increasing your physical activity is one of the best investments you can make for your future. Regular exercise can improve your health in many ways, including the following areas:

- Cardiovascular
- Gastrointestinal
- Immune System/Infections
- Mental/Neurologic
- Metabolic
- Musculoskeletal
- Pulmonary

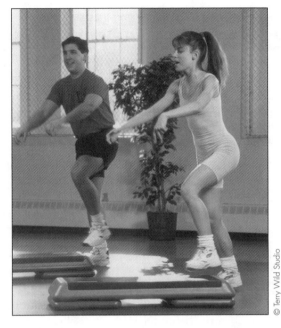

© Terry Wild Studio

work colleagues, or friends), they can encourage and support your participation in the fitness program.

3. *Emphasis on enjoyment.* Learning new behaviors must be pleasurable if you are to discard old behaviors. Choose an upbeat fitness program and activities with an enjoyable atmosphere. The performance approach (e.g., military or athletic) aimed only at producing results at the risk of hating the exercise will not work in a lifelong fitness program. Think about the potential fitness gains due to your new behavior rather than any negative aspects. Your contract with a friend or helper should focus on these gains through activities you enjoy.

4. *Quality programs.* Qualified and enthusiastic personnel; regular assessment of important fitness components; relevant personal and general communication; and a variety of group/individual exercises, games, and sports that interest you are all qualities of a good fitness program. Physical activity and socialization make a profitable combination, as evidenced by the success of many dance and physical fitness groups. Many people enjoy the social interaction with others who often support them in continuing the exercise.

5. *Role models.* People learn from each other and from others they admire. Choose a fitness instructor who displays healthy behaviors and enjoys a healthy lifestyle.

Table 2.2

Sample Contract to Begin Exercise

I, _____, do agree with _____ that I will begin the following
    (your name)   (helper's name)
walking program as of January 1, 2000:

1. I will walk from 7:00 to 7:30 A.M. on Monday, Wednesday, and Friday of each week.

2. I will record in writing my walking distance covered and comments on a weekly form.

3. I will take this form to _____ each Sunday afternoon and discuss any
                      (helper's name)
   problems I had as we walk together at 5:00 P.M.

4. In May, I will join the Plainview Fitness Center and attend a Tuesday–Thursday fitness
   class of my choice, continuing my Sunday afternoon walks with _____.
                                                (helper's name)

I will reward myself with the purchase of one new cassette each week of perfect attendance in
my program. At the end of each month of perfect attendance, I will buy a new compact disc of
my choice. At the end of each year of perfect attendance, I will treat my helper and myself to a
Broadway show in New York.

For each exercise session I miss, I will send a $25 contribution to the person who in my opinion
is the most hypocritical politician.

_____	_____	_____
(Signed)	(Date)	(Witness)

Reprinted, by permission, from B.D. Franks and E.T. Howley, 1998, *Fitness Leader's Handbook*, 2d ed.
(Champaign, IL: Human Kinetics), 147.

Another way to begin exercising is to do it on your own. In this
case, signing a contract with a friend is a good way to begin. Table 2.2
shows an example of what such a contract might include. (Of course,
you should modify it to be just right for you.)

Smoking

There is little disagreement with the statement that smoking compro-
mises health. Ample data indicate that smoking is the largest avoid-
able cause of death in the United States. Through warning labels on
packages and in advertisements, virtually all U.S. citizens are now
aware of the dangers of smoking. Millions of people have quit smoking, but if you are a smoker, you know it is a difficult habit to break.

Reasons for Smoking

Remember, our first step in changing behavior is to analyze the problem. Perhaps a brief summary of some of the environments in which

people smoke will help you understand your own reasons. Many smokers start and continue the habit because of social pressures— they do it with friends or in certain situations. Others smoke to relax while solving a problem, during a work break, watching a game, or after dinner. When do you smoke? Who else is around? What are you feeling when you smoke?

The so-called "rewards" of smoking include a series of "highs" when nicotine reaches the brain a few seconds after inhaling. An addiction to smoking is similar to addiction to other drugs. You experience a "craving" for a cigarette, and withdrawal symptoms make it a habit resistant to change. But you can break the habit, as millions have done. Now is a good time to do it.

Stop-Smoking Plan

The following plan for stopping smoking includes preparation, cessation, and maintenance.

Stage 1: Preparation

You need to gain confidence that you can succeed in quitting smoking. Foster your self-confidence by setting clear goals and determining procedures to follow. During the first stage, monitor your frequency of smoking. This self-observation often helps to reduce your smoking behavior temporarily.

Stage 2: Cessation

Ending the smoking behavior abruptly has been found to be more effective than gradually cutting down. An effective method to stop smoking is to sign a contract to quit on a specific date. The contract should involve a specific agreement between you and another person and should be very precise and linked to a specific time constraint. For example: "No cigarette will be smoked by Sheila Smith between the dates of December 31, 1999, and January 1, 2001." The contract should also specify the consequences if the contract is broken. For example, if Sheila Smith is a conservative Republican, her contract might stipulate that for each cigarette she smokes in 2000 she will send a $100 contribution to a liberal Democratic senator she particularly dislikes.

The contract should be individually tailored to your capabilities and needs. How long do you have to refrain from smoking to feel that you have quit? To whom can you send a donation to make the penalty especially aversive? What amount of money will help you abide by the conditions of the contract? Write into your contract any contingencies that will help you abide by the conditions of the contract. You will need frequent contact with your cosigner during the early part of the contract for encouragement and discussion of unanticipated problems. Table 2.3 outlines a sample contract that can be modified to fit your situation.

Stage 3: Maintenance

Once again, an old joke makes a good point: "Stopping smoking is easy—I've done it hundreds of times!" The real problem, of course, is to keep from starting to smoke again once you have quit. Maintaining contact with your helper and developing new behavioral skills are essential ingredients in maintaining the behavioral change. Remind yourself of the advantages of a smokeless life (e.g., lower risk of major health problems, less stress in daily activities).

You may have to learn new skills for dealing with old stimuli that you associate with smoking. If drinking coffee at the end of a meal was an old cue to light up, then perhaps avoiding coffee and drinking

Table 2.3
Sample Contract to Stop Smoking

I, _____, do agree with _____ to the following:
  (your name)   (helper's name)

1. Stop smoking as of 6:00 A.M., January 1, 2000.

2. I will call my helper each night at 7:00 P.M. during January, every Thursday night from February through May, and on the first of each month starting in June. We will discuss the problems I have had since our last call and set a time to meet if I need to talk with her in person.

3. During January, I will do the following at those times when, based on my past experience, I am most tempted to smoke:
   (a) Rub my pet rock with my right hand while talking with friends at social affairs
   (b) Eat fruit following dinner each night
   (c) Play a game of solitaire prior to going to sleep each night

I will reward myself with the purchase of one new cassette each week that I go without smoking. At the end of each smokeless month, I will buy a new compact disc of my choice. At the end of one year without smoking, I will treat my helper and myself to a Broadway show in New York.

For each cigarette I smoke during the year, I will send a $25 contribution to the person who in my opinion is the most hypocritical politician.

| _____ | _____ | _____ |
| (Signed) | (Date) | (Witness) |

Reprinted, by permission, from B.D. Franks and E.T. Howley, 1998, *Fitness Leader's Handbook*, 2d ed. (Champaign, IL: Human Kinetics), 148.

tea instead may eliminate that cue. If cigarette smoke in the lobby of a basketball arena during halftime provided a cue for lighting up, then either remaining seated in the arena or chewing gum in the lobby might be a new behavior. Once again we emphasize the importance of enlisting the support of others.

Alcohol Consumption

Alcoholism is one of our nation's leading public health problems. It is estimated that there are between 5 and 15 million alcoholics in the United States. The problems of family disruption, lost time at work, bodily injury, and death that are directly and indirectly due to excessive drinking are not disputed even by the producers of alcoholic beverages. Alcoholism exacts a heavy toll on the health and financial well-being of Americans.

Although there is no debate on the reality of the alcoholism problem, debate on appropriate goals for treating the problem is heated. Should an alcoholic strive for controlled moderate drinking or complete abstinence? Those who feel that abstinence is the correct goal tend to conceptualize the problem as a disease. The successful treatment approach of Alcoholics Anonymous (AA) is based on the disease concept. One fundamental precept of AA is that a person who has the disease of alcoholism will always have it—there is no cure. Combating the disease requires total abstinence. Alcoholics Anonymous helps individuals to achieve this goal with the support of other alcoholics via person-to-person contacts and regular group meetings.

Others contend that alcoholism is not a disease and that no crucial difference distinguishes the social drinker from the problem drinker besides the amount of alcohol consumed. Four factors that determine whether an individual will indulge in excessive drinking have been proposed: (1) the degree to which the individual feels controlled, (2) the availability of an adequate coping response, (3) expectations about the results of the drinking, and (4) the availability of alcohol and situational constraints. For example, (1) at a New

Even one shot decreases cognitive functions. Alcohol induces serious hypoglycemia, which is one of the main reasons for accidents and abnormal behavior.

Year's Eve party, you may feel strong pressure to drink; (2) you may not have an adequate coping response—you may feel uncomfortable asking for a soft drink and request liquor instead; (3) you may have pleasant memories of previous New Year's Eve parties that included excessive drinking; and (4) plenty of alcohol is available, and party-goers are expected to consume it.

Abstinence or Controlled Drinking

You must decide which choice is appropriate for you. In general, someone with a history of chronic alcohol abuse who has developed serious life problems associated with drinking may be more suited to the complete abstinence approach. A younger person who is open to learning new social skills may respond well to the controlled drinking approach. A contract similar to the one for stopping smoking (table 2.3) can be modified to help you either quit or control your drinking.

Controlled Drinking

If you believe you can control your drinking, then several suggestions may help you. Social skills training to reduce excessive drinking normally includes instruction in assertive response, refusing alcohol, relapse prevention, and ways to obtain reinforcement other than from drinking. In assertiveness training you learn how to communicate your feelings in a productive, caring manner. This type of training may help you if your excessive drinking behavior is related to an inability to communicate feelings to intimates and other associates. Learning how to refuse alcoholic drinks is also important. Some alcoholics simply lack practice in refusing a drink.

Many techniques can help you to abstain or drink less for a given period of time. However, it is difficult to maintain these improvements over a long period of time. Relapse prevention is probably the most important component of the social skills training plan. One of the key elements in maintaining the desired behavior is to be able to anticipate problem situations. Planning ways to avoid problems before the problems actually arise can help you discover behaviors other than excessive drinking that can provide positive reinforcement from your peers and important others. For example, improving your conversation or storytelling skills can give you a substitute for excessive drinking in some situations. You can use role-playing to avoid relapses. Discussing your feelings and coping behaviors in potential problem situations with a helper can be very helpful.

Weight Control

Obesity seems to be more difficult to overcome than either smoking or problem drinking. Fewer than 5 percent of obese individuals successfully lose weight and maintain their new weight, whereas 20 to 25 percent of smokers and alcoholics report success at quitting smoking or alcohol abuse. One problem seems to be an emphasis on "negative change" goals rather than on developing healthy substitute behaviors, for example, concentrating on eating less cheese rather than focusing on eating fruit at snack time.

Another problem in maintaining desired weight is a disregard for either energy intake or energy expenditure. Both decreased caloric intake and increased exercise (caloric expenditure) are normally essential for maintaining desired weight. Disregarding either one dooms most people to failure.

Efforts to control weight can be thwarted by direct attacks on eating behavior rather than on the indirect reasons for the behavior. If a particular cue results in poor eating behavior, it can help to either avoid the cue or learn to react to it differently. The ready access of food and drink and media messages promoting a relationship between happiness and what you consume contribute to the problems people have in trying to change their eating behaviors.

Chapter 3 deals with methods of determining percent fat and estimating ideal weight. It is important that you work toward your goal gradually in ways that you can accept physiologically and psychologically.

Weight Loss

No single weight-loss program can be recommended for everyone. Much of your success depends on you deciding what steps are likely to work for you. The following seven components, however, appear to be common ingredients in all successful programs.

1. *Self-monitoring.* Before you implement any specific steps, keep a daily diary for two weeks describing the quantity of food you eat and your eating environments.

2. *Treatment goals.* Once you determine your ideal weight goal, perhaps in consultation with a fitness leader, set weekly goals (from one-half to two pounds per week). If you are extremely obese (greater than 40 percent fat if female, greater than 30 percent fat if male), seek medical supervision.

3. *Diet selection.* Select a dietary plan that specifies food type, portions, and calorie amounts. You may want to use the Food Guide Pyramid outlined in chapter 4.

4. *Stimulus control.* Certain situations or cues are often strongly related to eating patterns (e.g., watching a movie or television). Decide to eat only in certain places (e.g., the dining room table, the cafeteria at work) and only at certain times (e.g., breakfast, lunch, supper, and one snack time).

5. *Self-reward.* Some people are helped by giving themselves small rewards for progress toward their goals (e.g., a new audiotape for each three-pound loss) and a larger reward (e.g., tickets to a Broadway show) when they reach the final goal. The rewards should be consistent with healthy behaviors, something you enjoy, and things for which there are no acceptable alternatives.

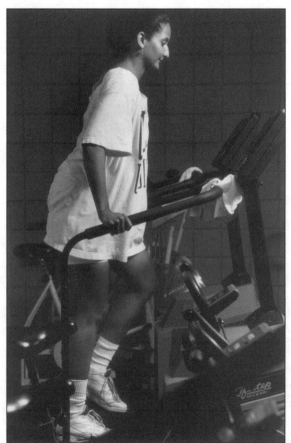

© Terry Wild Studio

6. *Exercise.* The first section of this chapter dealt with ways to begin and continue regular exercise. Although everyone who begins an exercise program does not necessarily need to begin a weight-loss program, most people who need to lose fat should begin diet and exercise programs simultaneously. People who are physically active are more likely to maintain a desired weight once they have achieved it.

7. *Support.* The support of a spouse or other important person can greatly assist you in staying with the program. The involvement of friends or family members early in the program enhances the probability of its success.

Stress

Chapter 9 addresses the issues of stress in greater depth. For now, simply pay attention to your interaction with potential stressors as a way to reduce excessive stress. The three stages of stress reduction are preparation, skill acquisition, and practice. You can go through them by yourself, but you may find it helpful to work with a fitness leader or counselor.

1. The first stage involves preparing yourself mentally for a coming stressful situation. Keep a diary of the frequency of and conditions surrounding the stressor.

2. In the skill acquisition stage, the main emphasis is on learning basic cognitive and behavioral coping skills. One of the skills is "private speech," in which you rehearse sentences to say to yourself prior to, during, and following the stressor. For example, prior to a major test or presentation of a report, you may tell yourself, "It's going to be hard, but I have prepared for it." During the event you may say, "If I stay calm I will be less likely to block on a question," and/or "I'm getting tense—relax and take it easy." Following the event you may tell yourself, "I did as well as I could because I stayed calm."

A second component of the skill acquisition stage is relaxation training. Chapter 9 outlines a procedure of tensing and relaxing specific muscle groups. With practice, you can rapidly achieve a relaxed state in a potentially stressful situation.

3. In the final, or practice, stage, you set up a series of practice situations that help you learn to apply the previously taught skills. The situations should progress from mildly stressful to more severely stressful so that you can experience success and gain confidence in using the skills.

One of the primary objectives of a fitness program is to help participants modify lifestyle behaviors. Although the focus of attention is on increasing exercise, it should be clear that unhealthy behaviors need to be decreased. The following guidelines can help you change unhealthy behaviors.

- Analyze the history of the problem and record the current status of the behavior.
- Set a long-term goal and several short-term goals, and sign a contract with a friend.
- List as many strategies as possible to resolve the problem, selecting one or two that will be most effective.
- Learn new coping skills and have regular meetings with a helper.
- Once you reach the goal, outline a maintenance schedule that includes periodic contacts with your helper.

Taking control of your life by recognizing and changing unhealthy behaviors puts you well on the road to total fitness.

chapter 3

Controlling Your Weight

Many Americans have a full-time preoccupation with losing weight. This is due partly to social pressure to have a certain "look" and partly to the health consequences of carrying too much fat. People who are too fat are more likely to have high blood pressure, heart disease, and diabetes. The purpose of this chapter is to help you separate fact from fiction with regard to body composition and weight control.

Analyzing Your Weight

A variety of weight-to-height tables have been used over the years to classify a person as being overweight or underweight by comparing the person's body weight to that of people of the same gender and height. One central problem with these tables is that they do not distinguish between a person who is heavily muscled from weightlifting and someone who is fat due in part to a sedentary lifestyle. In spite of these limitations, these indexes can be useful because so many individuals fall into the sedentary category.

One of the most common of these weight-to-height ratios is the body mass index (BMI). The BMI is the ratio of the person's weight (in kilograms) to height (in meters) squared (kg/m^2). Table 3.1 can be used to find your BMI. Find the row with your height in inches and the column with your weight in pounds—where they intersect is your BMI. For example, an individual who is 65 inches tall and weighs 120 pounds has a BMI of 20.0. The evaluation of your BMI is found at the bottom of table 3.1. In this example, the person has a good BMI.

Since the BMI does not provide information about body composition, other techniques are needed.

Components of Body Composition

The human body is composed of a wide variety of tissues and organs such as muscle, bone, fat, heart, liver, and brain. To simplify our discussion of body composition, we will divide the body into fat mass and fat-free mass and express each as a percent of total body weight. For example, a man who is 20 percent fat and weighs 200 pounds is carrying 40 pounds of fat (20 percent of 200 pounds). Fat-free mass includes all tissues and organs other than fat. Fat mass includes *essential fat* (fat that is necessary for survival) and the "extra" that we carry around.

Table 3.1

Body Mass Index (BMI)

	Weight (lbs)						
Ht. (in.)	110	120	130	140	150	160	170
60	21.5	23.5	25.4	27.4	29.3	31.3	33.2
61	20.8	22.7	24.6	26.5	28.4	30.3	32.1
62	20.1	22.0	23.8	25.6	27.5	29.3	31.1
63	19.5	21.3	23.0	24.8	26.6	28.4	30.1
64	18.9	20.6	22.3	24.1	25.8	27.5	29.2
65	18.3	20.0	21.7	23.3	25.0	26.6	28.3
66	17.8	19.4	21.0	22.6	24.2	25.8	27.5
67	17.2	18.8	20.4	21.9	23.5	25.1	26.6
68	16.7	18.3	19.8	21.3	22.8	24.3	25.9
69	16.3	17.7	19.2	20.7	22.2	23.6	25.1
70	15.8	17.2	18.7	20.1	21.5	23.0	24.4
71	15.4	16.8	18.1	19.5	20.9	22.3	23.7
72	14.9	16.3	17.6	19.0	20.4	21.7	23.1
73	14.5	15.8	17.2	18.5	19.8	21.1	22.4
74	14.1	15.4	16.7	18.0	19.3	20.6	21.8
75	13.8	15.0	16.3	17.5	18.8	20.0	21.3
76	13.4	14.6	15.8	17.1	18.3	19.5	20.7
77	13.1	14.2	15.4	16.6	17.8	19.0	20.2
78	12.7	13.9	15.0	16.2	17.3	18.5	19.7

	Weight (lbs)						
Ht. (in.)	180	190	200	210	220	230	240
60	35.2	37.1	39.1	41.0	43.0	45.0	46.9
61	34.0	35.9	37.8	39.7	41.6	43.5	45.4
62	33.0	34.8	36.6	38.4	40.3	42.1	43.9
63	31.9	33.7	35.5	37.2	39.0	40.8	42.6
64	30.9	32.6	34.4	36.1	37.8	39.5	41.2
65	30.0	31.6	33.3	35.0	36.6	38.3	40.0
66	29.1	30.7	32.3	33.9	35.5	37.2	38.8
67	28.2	29.8	31.4	32.9	34.5	36.1	37.6
68	27.4	28.9	30.4	32.0	33.5	35.0	36.5
69	26.6	28.1	29.6	31.0	32.5	34.0	35.5
70	25.9	27.3	28.7	30.2	31.6	33.0	34.5
71	25.1	26.5	27.9	29.3	30.7	32.1	33.5
72	24.4	25.8	27.1	28.5	29.9	31.2	32.6
73	23.8	25.1	26.4	27.7	29.1	30.4	31.7
74	23.1	24.4	25.7	27.0	28.3	29.6	30.8
75	22.5	23.8	25.0	26.3	27.5	28.8	30.0
76	21.9	23.1	24.4	25.6	26.8	28.0	29.2
77	21.4	22.6	23.7	24.9	26.1	27.3	28.5
78	20.8	22.0	23.1	24.3	25.4	26.6	27.8

20–24.9 = Good
25–27   = Borderline
> 27   = Risk of health problems

Fat is found in all cells, surrounds most nerves, and is associated with specific tissues. Essential fat totals about 3 to 5 percent of body weight for men and 11 to 14 percent of body weight for women. The higher value for women allows for the fat that is usually deposited in the breasts and hips at puberty and is related to the hormone estrogen. Understanding the nature of essential fat is important because it sets the lower limit of body fatness for men and women.

What, then, is a reasonable amount of fat? Does it matter where it is located (e.g., hips or abdomen)? Healthy body fatness values are neither too low nor too high. In the past, most fitness books were concerned solely with too much fat; that is no longer true. Our country has experienced an increased incidence of eating disorders as some people (primarily teenage girls and young women) strive to be as thin as possible. *Anorexia nervosa* is an eating disorder in which people have a distorted view of their body fatness; they see themselves as fat even if they are emaciated. *Bulimia* describes a ritual of overeating followed by vomiting to help keep body weight low. Concern about these eating disorders has led to the identification of both low and high body fatness values that are consistent with good health.

Recommended body fatness values will be different for the athlete interested in world-class performance than for the average person participating in a health-related fitness program. Figure 3.1 lists body fatness values that bracket the healthy range. Your goal should be to achieve that optimal range. Keep in mind the fact that body fatness normally fluctuates some amount during the year as physical activity and food consumption patterns vary with the seasons and holidays.

Tests of Body Fatness

Body fatness can be evaluated by a wide variety of techniques; this section will address only the most common. We will start by excluding some, then recommending others.

The "mirror test," in which you stand naked in front of a full-length mirror, requires strict objectivity to discern what is too fat and what is too thin. Although it is not a bad idea to take a look at ourselves in this way every once in a while, we can sometimes fool ourselves into thinking we are just right when we are in fact fat or thinking we are too fat when we are actually very thin, as in the case of anorexia nervosa.

One recommended way to analyze body composition is *underwater weighing*, also known as hydrostatic weighing, which measures

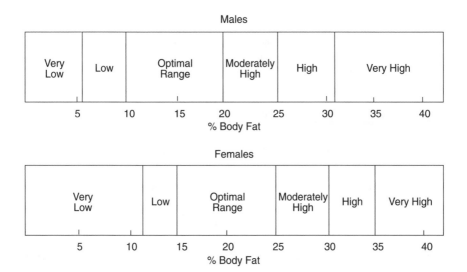

Figure 3.1 Body fatness values

This article figure is reprinted with permission from *The Journal of Physical Education, Recreation & Dance,* September, 1987, pp. 98–102. *JOPERD* is a publication of the American Alliance for Health, Physical Education, Recreation and Dance, 1900 Association Drive, Reston, VA 20191.

body density or the tendency of a person to sink in water. With this technique, your weight is measured on land with a calibrated scale and again when you are completely submerged in water. The idea is that, because fat tends to float, a lean person will weigh more underwater than a fat person of the same weight will. For example, if we measured the underwater weight of two people, each weighing 200 pounds, the person with the lower body density would weigh less. On the basis of the land and underwater weights, the density and relative fatness of the body are calculated. This technique is accurate but time consuming, and doing it correctly requires special equipment and personnel. This makes it an expensive way to determine body fatness, and it is not commonly used.

The most common method of evaluating body composition is by measuring the thickness of several skinfolds. Because a large amount of total body fat is located just under the skin, overall body fatness can be estimated by estimating that fat.

If you are in a good fitness program, you have probably had your percent fat estimated by underwater weighing or skinfold measurements. If you are not in a fitness program and want to determine your percent fat and how much you should lose or gain, check with a fitness program or personal fitness trainer in your area. You will know, of course, that your fat levels are changing when you notice that your clothes fit differently.

Distribution of Body Fat

Individuals who store a large portion of their body fat in the trunk area ("apple-shaped obesity") have a higher risk of heart disease and diabetes than those who carry the fat on the hips and buttocks ("pear-shaped obesity"). A simple measurement to evaluate the degree to which you are shaped like an apple or a pear is the *waist-to-hip ratio.* Women with values above .86 and men with values above .95 are at a high risk of developing these diseases. To measure the waist-to-hip ratio, use the following procedure:

1. Wear little clothing, allowing the tape to be placed at the proper location.
2. Stand in front of a mirror and place the measuring tape around the narrowest part of your torso, between the umbilicus (belly button) and the bottom of the sternum (breast bone). Keep the tape parallel to the ground. Record in centimeters or inches.
3. Place the tape around your buttocks where it is the largest. Keep the tape parallel to the ground and measure in centimeters or inches.
4. Divide the measurement in step 2 by the measurement in step 3. For example, if a male has a waist circumference of 96.5 cm (38 in.) and a hip circumference of 99.1 cm (39 in.), then his waist-to-hip ratio is .97 and he is at a high risk of developing cardiovascular and metabolic disease.

Target Weight

We encourage you to have your percent fat determined by underwater weighing or by skinfold site measurements by fitness professionals. You can then determine your desired weight using that estimated percent fat. This is a better way of deciding your optimal weight than simply using a height/weight chart because this method is based on how much fat you should have.

1. Weigh yourself to get your current body weight: _____ pounds

2. Record the percent body fat: _____ percent

3. Multiply your percent body fat, converted to a decimal value, by your body weight to yield fat weight in pounds:

   Percent body fat (._____) times body weight (____pounds) equals _____ pounds of fat weight

4. Subtract this fat weight from your total body weight to yield fat-free body weight:

   Body weight (_____ pounds) minus fat weight (_____ pounds) equals ____ pounds fat-free weight

5. Divide fat-free weight by .80 to .90 (allowing for 10 to 20 percent ideal body fatness for men), or by .75 to .85 (15 to 25 percent body fat for women). This is the target weight range.

For example:

1. If a man is 24 percent fat and weighs 189 pounds, his fat weight is 45.4 pounds (.24 times 189 pounds equals 45.4 pounds).

2. Subtracting 45.4 pounds from 189 pounds leaves 143.6 pounds for fat-free body weight.

3. His ideal body fatness range is 10 to 20 percent, so divide 143.6 pounds by .80 and 143.6 pounds by .90 to yield 160 to 180 pounds as his target weight range.

4. He should try to achieve the upper part of the target weight range at a rate of one pound every two weeks (in this example, a loss of 9 pounds from 189 to 180 within 18 weeks).

Changing Your Fat Level

The previous sections described the difference between body weight and body fat. This section deals with the issues related to changing body weight and body composition.

Caloric Balance and Weight Control

When we discuss weight control and body composition, we are dealing with the issues of *gaining and losing fat and lean tissue.* There is no question that body weight can be lost through excessive sweating

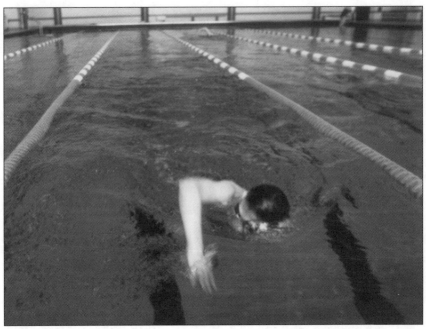

© Terry Wild Studio

or with the use of diuretic drugs that cause the kidneys to produce lots of urine. However, water weight is easily replaced and has no effect on fat weight. Therefore, in our discussion of this topic we will refer only to methods that alter the fat mass and the lean mass of the body, thus altering body composition to improve health status.

Caloric intake refers to the number of kilocalories (kcal)—called simply *calories* in everyday usage—of food consumed. Calorie expenditure is related to the following:

- Resting metabolic rate—the amount of energy you use while lying or sitting. What may surprise you is that resting metabolic rate represents about 60 to 70 percent of a person's total daily energy expenditure. The resting metabolic rate is directly related to the fat-free mass.

- Physical activity associated with work, recreation, and sports represents about 20 to 30 percent of daily energy expenditure. This is the area in which your daily choices can help you in maintaining your desirable weight.

- Thermic effect of food—the amount of energy required to process the food you eat. This equals about 10 percent of total daily energy expenditure.

ENERGY BALANCE EQUATION

The central concept related to weight control is found in the *energy balance equation*:

If caloric intake *is equal to* caloric expenditure, then energy balance exists—no change in weight occurs.

If caloric intake *is greater than* caloric expenditure, then positive energy balance exists—weight gain occurs.

If caloric intake *is less than* caloric expenditure, then negative energy balance exists—weight loss occurs.

Chapter 5 provides estimates of daily caloric expenditures for different activity levels. To maintain your body weight you must balance caloric intake and expenditure, and *if you wish to lose weight you must create a negative energy balance by expending more calories than you consume.*

This negative energy balance can be accomplished by keeping your energy expenditure the same and reducing your caloric intake. In this case, the focus of attention is on trying to eat a nutritionally sound diet while consuming fewer calories (see chapter 4). You can also lose weight by keeping your diet the same but increasing your energy expenditure. In either case, you must lose 3,500 calories from your body's energy store to lose one pound of fat. If you were to create a negative energy balance of 500 calories per day, you would lose about one pound of fat per week. The recommended rate of weight loss is a *maximum* of two pounds per week, so the total negative energy balance should be no more than about 1,000 calories per day. We recommend more modest changes in diet and exercise to achieve a loss of one pound every two weeks.

Diet and Exercise

Even though you can lose weight by diet or exercise, for reasons explained below, we recommend that you use a combination of the two to achieve your goal.

• When you reduce your caloric intake, your body responds as if you are beginning to starve. One of the body's adaptations is to decrease the resting metabolic rate to save the body's energy stores. This means that a diet very low in calories can become counterproductive to weight loss; the more you cut back on caloric intake, the more the body responds by decreasing its energy expenditure.

• When you lose weight by diet alone, 35 to 45 percent of the weight lost is lean tissue, not fat tissue. Therefore, you could actually lose weight but not change your percent of body fatness (body composition) very much. This loss of lean tissue also contributes to the body's reduction in resting metabolic rate, making it more difficult for you to lose weight. Resistance training (see chapter 7) can increase muscle mass and help maintain the resting metabolic rate.

A weight-loss program that uses diet alone results in a slower rate of fat loss. It should be no surprise, then, that a combination of diet and exercise is recommended to achieve weight-loss and body-composition goals. Exercise helps to maintain lean muscle tissue and the resting metabolic rate while more fat is being lost; the body actually makes changes in percent body fat faster than it can through diet alone. We have seen many cases in which body weight may not change for several weeks but clothing sizes do. Why does this hap-

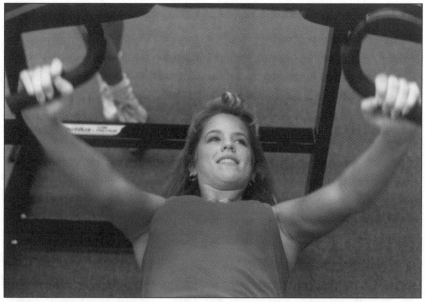

© Terry Wild Studio

pen? The exercise is increasing lean body mass while fat mass is decreasing slightly. With time, body weight will decrease in proportion to the change in energy balance.

Exercise and Weight Management

In the following paragraphs we discuss some facts about exercise and weight loss. We also present information that should prove to you that exercise is a very beneficial part of your lifestyle, whether you are losing weight or not.

The body expends energy whether at rest, work, or play. A person must take in and use oxygen (O_2) for this to occur. In fact, if we know how much oxygen is being used, we can calculate how many calories of energy the body expends. The body's use of one liter of oxygen causes the expenditure of five calories of energy. This is a very important point in understanding the role of exercise in weight loss.

We have already indicated that a negative caloric balance of 3,500 calories is necessary to lose one pound of fat tissue. For example, imagine there are two people trying to lose weight—one by sitting in a sauna and the other by running around a track. The person sitting in the sauna expends only 72 calories per hour because the body uses very little oxygen while sitting at rest. The person running around the track, however, expends about 600 calories per hour because the body requires a great deal of oxygen to run. To expend the caloric equivalent of one pound of fat (3,500 calories), it would take 50 hours of sitting in a sauna but only 6 hours of running.

Fortunately, you do not have to do all that exercise at one time! Remember, a combination of diet and exercise will result in a steady reduction in body weight and leave you with diet and activity habits you can accept as part of your lifestyle. See chapter 5 for a discussion of the caloric costs of various activities.

Exercise and Appetite

You might think that if you exercise more you will eat more, lessening the effect of your exercise on your weight. People who begin moderate exercise programs, however, show little or no change in appetite. Most people can do fitness workouts of 30 to 60 minutes several days a week without increasing their caloric intake. Some individuals even find that they are not as hungry and eat less when they are active on a regular basis.

Diet, Exercise, and Cholesterol

Proper exercise and diet affect more than weight. Research has shown that a low-fat diet that contains 30 percent or less of calories from fat (such as the one discussed in chapter 4) is associated with low levels of serum cholesterol, one of the major risk factors of heart disease. In addition, exercise appears to have a separate effect of raising the level of "good" high-density lipoprotein cholesterol (HDL-C). Lowering total cholesterol and raising HDL-C reduces the risk of heart disease.

Once you have analyzed your body composition and distribution of body fat, you are in a position to determine your target weight and plan a fitness program to achieve it. Through a combination of diet and exercise, you can attain your target weight while improving your health status in the process.

chapter 4

Eating Healthily

A s a society, we have a love-hate relationship with food. Two of the best-selling types of books are those dealing with cooking and dieting. Good nutrition is essential for optimal health. Poor eating habits are a major cause of many health problems. This chapter will give you the basic facts and reasonable alternatives regarding what you should (and should not) do in your own food selection, but we start by helping you understand the broader context of how nutrition has evolved in human history.

Our relationship to food has changed dramatically from that of our earliest ancestors. Like other primates, our ancestors were herbivores, feeding on leaves, roots, seeds, and fruits. Because the foraging and grazing necessary for survival required them to travel long distances, food was clearly the most important part of their existence.

Later, as humans learned to cultivate land and raise and store crops, food became a trading commodity and was used in a social/religious context in celebrations and offerings. As the availability of food increased, eating habits changed too. Although eating meats became more possible with the discovery of primitive tools and firearms, it became more regular with the domestication of animals that happened during nomadic times, long before first settlements. However, grains, vegetables, and fruits dominated our diets long after settlements up to modern times when the influence of commercialism surpassed that of education.

Interestingly, like other herbivores (e.g., sheep, monkeys) our intestines are much longer than the intestines of mammals that feed on flesh (carnivores) and gorge themselves at feedings (e.g., dogs, wolves). Although carnivores have shorter intestines and feed mainly on protein and fat, they rarely develop arteriosclerosis, coronary heart disease, or stroke as humans do. This is due to their active lives as predators and their gorging, which is a way of fattening up to survive long fasts during lean periods (e.g., winters in the north or the dry summers of Africa). In other words, their eating habits are related to their climates, environments, and active lifestyles—all of which change in captivity (e.g., a zoo), making them prone to cardiovascular disease in such settings.

Proteins and fats need a long time for digestion. Therefore, their digestion and absorption are enhanced in the long intestines of humans. Carnivores have a large meal (gorge) when they catch their prey and then rest for quite a while, sometimes for days. This is because after a large meal consisting of fat and protein, the body reduces blood flow for all other activities/systems, including muscles, and diverts it to the digestive tract. Humans, too, often feel exhausted and want to rest after a large meal. This is not observed after a small meal, especially one consisting of vegetables. Thus, resuming exercise two to three hours after meals will allow sufficient blood for digestion and eliminate the gastrointestinal problems such as cramps and nausea that may occur during exercise immediately after meals.

Large studies undertaken in Africa revealed that rural and nomadic people who foraged frequently did not exhibit the diseases such as hypertension, cardiovascular problems, and diabetes that their fellow tribesmen experienced after moving to cities. Generally speaking, herbivores eat small amounts frequently and live longer, whereas carnivores eat huge amounts, although less frequently, but live shorter lives. In short, our biological heritage is more consistent with that of herbivores who forage for carbohydrates than that of carnivores who gorge on fats and protein. Humans can leave nature but nature will never leave them.

Eating habits and foods vary according to lifestyles. Putting aside ancient history, the eating habits of people only 50 years ago were quite different from ours. In the South, for example, people used to work in the cotton fields very early in the morning to escape the scorching sun. They usually had one large meal (usually deep fried and rich in fat) early in the afternoon. Fats are the richest source of calories (nine calories per gram) and provide the most satiety. Such eating practices are still observed in similar working conditions all around the world. Thus, the common practice of three meals a day is not necessarily a physiological requirement but rather an innovation of urbanization and industrialization.

The appearance of food, its presentation and color, and our sense of smell and taste all play an important role in inducing a feeling of hunger and increasing appetite. Like other primates, our ancestors used their sense of smell to locate food. Herbs and spices were later used to preserve food and increase its palatability. Now they are sometimes used for the sole purpose of increasing consumption.

Much of the food advertised on television is not healthy, and most food-marketing campaigns are aimed at children who spend a lot of time watching TV. In addition, much of our food is processed, containing unhealthy preservatives and artificial colors. Some of the factors contributing to our nutritional problems are the ready availability and aggressive marketing of unhealthy food.

The metabolism of glucose varies from person to person. Daily variations of blood glucose levels are said to be as unique for each person as fingerprints. This implies that people do not have to eat the same number of meals at the same times. Some people may need only two meals a day, whereas others may need multiple snacks during the day.

When we wait until we are very hungry to eat, we often overeat (gorge) simple and processed sugars. This induces a larger than usual secretion of insulin, which in turn brings down the glucose level faster than usual, even to hypoglycemic levels, causing postprandial hypoglycemia (low blood glucose after eating). Hypoglycemia is not only linked to weakness or fainting but also mimics a variety of psychological and neurological problems. Authorities therefore recommend that we eat before blood sugar levels are so low that gorging becomes uncontrollable. They also recommend complex or natural carbohydrates instead of simple or processed sugars.

Our eating habits are strongly influenced by our mental status. When eating becomes an outlet for frustrations and a ritual to deal with depression, it can be as addictive as drinking or smoking. We tend to eat more when we are happy and when we are sad; some express their psychological problems by binge-eating, others with anorexia. Eating disorders once observed only among upper middle class young women are now becoming prevalent in men and other age groups. Eating accompanied by alcoholic beverages has become an important vehicle for socialization. Calories are lavishly gained on dates, at business dinners, at birthday parties, during "happy hours," and even at funerals.

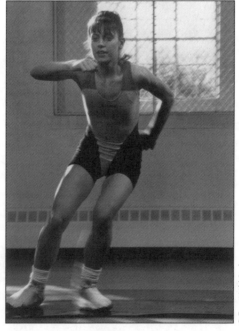

© Terry Wild Studio

Herbal Drugs and Ergogenic Aids

When European physicians landed in the Americas during the colonization period, they were overwhelmed by the thousands of inexpensive remedies available and an army of indigenous healers. Instead of studying the existing system's benefits and building on it, however, they chose to abolish it, establishing a professional health care system as a distinct entity isolated from communities.

Nevertheless, certain herbal extracts (e.g., digitalis, belladonna alkaloids, quinine, ephedrine, capsicum) that have been known for thousands of years are still being used effectively in today's professional medical practices. The inadequacy, poor accessibility, and expense of health care in modern societies seem to be the most important factors in creating a huge herbal drug industry, which is now worth billions. However, the most common users of these drugs are educated Caucasians with an annual income of over $35,000.

Because native people used only the actual plants or certain parts of plants, their toxic effects were minimized. Now, through processing, concentrating, and synthesizing the active ingredients of those same plants, the healing, as well as toxic, properties of the plants are heightened.

Coca leaves were used for a variety of ailments for centuries without any of the deadly effects observed currently. The cocaine snorted by addicts today is highly concentrated and much more potent than the coca leaves. It abruptly increases blood pressure to extreme levels that lead to stroke, the main cause of death in cocaine intoxication. Many herbal drugs can have serious toxic effects when used in high concentrations. Some of them are hallucinogens (e.g., jimsonweed), sedatives (e.g., kava kava, valerian), and stimulants (e.g., ginseng). Some herbal teas (e.g., bush tea) are toxic to the liver.

Research into the benefits of herbal drugs has increased as a result of their popularity. One recent study of echinacea, one of the most commonly advertised herbal drugs, did not find it to boost the immune system at all, as is claimed. Other studies have found gingko and St. John's wort to ameliorate depression and palmetto products to benefit benign prosthetic hyperplasia.

Despite a lack of information on the long-term effects of herbal drugs, research studies are important in this era of aggressive marketing and advertising, which even includes prescription medicine. Public distrust and increased scrutiny of the advertising industry has increased in the last few years as a result of aggressively marketed drugs being withdrawn from the market after serious complications were discovered.

What we have discussed under herbal drugs also applies to the so-called "ergogenic" aids to boost energy and build muscle mass. Taking drugs to enhance performance and pleasure is as old as history. However, the use of high doses of ergogenic aids and herbal drugs has reached such levels that it can only be considered drug abuse. For example, the overuse of anabolic steroids and growth hormone has serious and usually irreversible effects. Our addiction to such drugs should not be surprising in a society in which tobacco and liquor are lavishly, relentlessly, and very successfully advertised. The media and especially the entertainment industry, including professional sports, encourage the use of such drugs by behaving as if our only virtues are fun, pleasure, physical appearance, and performance.

Toll of Unhealthy Eating

Healthy eating involves more than just the proper amount of calories. This section will present some basic information on diet and healthy nutritional goals. We now have clear evidence that the typical American diet has adversely affected our health. For example, about 40 percent of our children are overweight. The overconsumption of saturated fats and the rate of heart disease in this country are clearly linked. In addition, excess body fat and the lack of dietary fiber have been tied to a variety of serious health problems. Recent research has linked many other diseases to nutritional risk factors.

Because of the high disease and death rates related to unhealthy eating, authorities have recommended important changes in our dietary habits. Table 4.1 summarizes these recommendations.

Eating Recommendations

The U.S. Departments of Agriculture (USDA) and Health and Human Services use the Food Guide Pyramid (figure 4.1) with the following dietary guidelines:

- Eat a variety of foods.
- Balance the food you eat with physical activity to maintain or improve your weight.

COSTS OF UNHEALTHY EATING

Following is a brief summary of diseases and conditions that have been linked to unhealthy eating and their cost in human life.

- Heart attacks: 1.5 million attacks and 520,000 deaths each year
- Cancers of colon, breast, and prostate: 130,000 deaths annually
- Hypertension: 58 million Americans
- Obesity (a risk factor for diabetes and hypertension): 32 million Americans aged 25–74
- Diabetes: 11 million Americans, contributes to 130,000 deaths each year
- Osteoporosis-related fractures: 1.3 million each year. Many are fatal hip fractures.
- Frequent constipation: 3.5 million Americans
- Intestinal diverticulosis: 1.5 million Americans
- Dental caries: an average of 8 cavities by age 9 and an average of 10–17 decayed or missing teeth among adults.

- Choose a diet
  - with plenty of grains, fruits and vegetables;
  - low in total fat, saturated fat, and cholesterol;
  - moderate in sodium; and
  - with a moderate amount of alcohol if you drink (one to two drinks every other day).

The base of the Food Guide Pyramid consists of carbohydrates (with 6 to 11 servings), and the top of the pyramid recommends limiting the use of fats, oils, sweets, and alcohol, all of which contribute little nutritional value to the diet while increasing the caloric content.

The Food Guide Pyramid suggested by the USDA has been challenged recently by the Mediterranean Diet prevalent in Spain, Italy, Greece, Turkey, and the North African coastline, where rates of cancer and heart disease are much lower than in the United States. Therefore, some nutritionists recommend this diet. Table 4.2 compares these two diets and the recently introduced DASH Diet for preventing and controlling high blood pressure.

Table 4.1

Current Practices and Recommendations for Daily Caloric Intake and Quantities* from Nutrients

Daily Quantity and % of Calories	Current Practice	Recommendation
Proteins	60+ g	60 g, 12%
Carbohydrates	45% of cal	55–60%
Complex	22% of cal	48%
Natural sugars	6% of cal	10%
Refined sugars	17% of cal	1–5%
Fiber	10–15 g	20–35 g
Fats	35–40% of cal	30% or less**
Saturated	16% of cal	5–10%
Monounsaturated	19% of cal	10+%
Polyunsaturated	7%	10% of cal
Cholesterol	450 mg	300 mg or less
Sodium	4–6 g	1–3 g

*1 gram (g) = 1,000 milligrams (mg); 1,000 g = 1 kilogram (kg) = 2.2 pounds
**Diets containing as little as 5–10% of calories as fat are safe. Current recommendations are to replace saturated fats with monounsaturated fats and complex carbohydrates.

The DASH Diet is based on 2,000 calories a day, but daily servings may vary according to energy needs. It is rich in vegetables and fruits and low in cholesterol and fats. This diet is also high in fiber, potassium, calcium, and magnesium and moderately high in protein. Diets deficient in potassium, calcium, and magnesium tend to increase blood pressure. Authorities suggest that the DASH Diet can be an effective strategy for everyone to prevent the increase in blood pressure with age and to reduce overall blood pressure levels. Some argue that the use of this diet throughout society may be more successful at decreasing cardiovascular disease and death in the general population than the current practice of simply providing treatment to those with the disease.

The Mediterranean Diet unfortunately does not specify servings for each type of food but only their intake frequency. It is similar to the DASH Diet with respect to fruits, vegetables, and grains. The main fat sources in the Mediterranean Diet are monounsaturated fatty acids, which decrease low-density cholesterol (LDL-C) and increase the de-

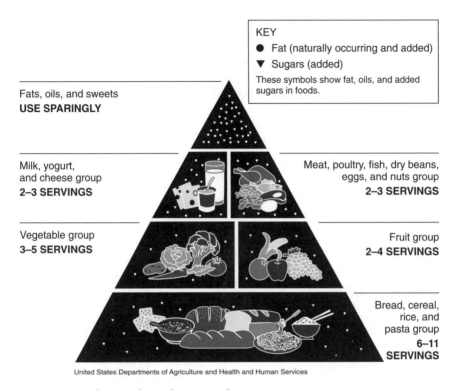

KEY
● Fat (naturally occurring and added)
▼ Sugars (added)
These symbols show fat, oils, and added sugars in foods.

Fats, oils, and sweets
USE SPARINGLY

Milk, yogurt, and cheese group
2–3 SERVINGS

Meat, poultry, fish, dry beans, eggs, and nuts group
2–3 SERVINGS

Vegetable group
3–5 SERVINGS

Fruit group
2–4 SERVINGS

Bread, cereal, rice, and pasta group
6–11 SERVINGS

United States Departments of Agriculture and Health and Human Services

Figure 4.1 The Food Guide Pyramid

sirable high-density cholesterol (HDL-C). Red wine, suggested in this diet, contains phenolic antioxidants, which decrease LDL-C and prevent clotting. However, an aspirin (80–300 mg) a day and several cups of tea can serve the same purpose. (The same reasoning applies to the recent news that beer contains flavonoids and can protect us from certain types of cancer. Citrus fruits, especially grapefruits, contain flavonoids without the adverse effects of alcohol.)

In order to understand the recommended amounts in any diet, we must be able to describe and quantify the servings. The following describes the amount for *one serving* of each food group:

Sweets, Fats, and Oils
   1 tsp

Proteins
   Meat servings should not exceed 3 oz
      1/2 cup cooked sliced meat
      1/2 chicken breast

Table 4.2

Comparison of USDA Guidelines
With the Mediterranean and DASH Diets

Foods	DAILY SERVINGS		Mediterranean Diet (weekly/daily frequency)
	USDA	DASH Diet*	
Fats, oils, and sweets	Use sparingly	0	No fats except olive oil (Daily); sweets (2–3/wk)
Milk, yogurt, cheese	2–3	2–3	Daily
Meat, poultry, fish, eggs	2–3	<2	2–3/wk, meat (Few times/month)
Nuts, dry beans	2–3	4–5/wk	Daily
Vegetables	3–5	4–5	Daily
Fruits	2–4	4–5	Daily
Bread, rice, cereal, pasta	6–11	7–8	Daily
1–2 oz. of red wine[a]	0	0	Daily

[a]One gram alcohol provides 7 calories. One serving provides 100–150 cal = 1-1/2 oz of hard liquor, 4 oz of wine, 12 oz of beer.
*DASH Diet servings are from the Dietary Approaches to Stop Hypertension clinical study: Based on data from The Sixth Report of the Joint National Committee on Prevention, Detection, Evaluation, and Treatment of High Blood Pressure. National Institutes of Health (Archives of Internal Medicine 157).

　　3 slices luncheon meat
　　1-1/2 cups cooked legumes (e.g., beans, peas, lentils)
　　3 eggs (weekly maximum)

Grains
　　1/4 cup granola cereal
　　1/2 cup pasta (cooked), bagel, or pita bread
　　2 cups puffed cereal
　　1 slice of bread, 1 pancake, or 4 crackers

Vegetables
　　1/2 cup sliced vegetables
　　1 cup leafy vegetables
　　1-1/2 cups mushrooms
　　1 six-inch ear of corn

Fruits
　　1/4 cup dried sliced fruit
　　1/2 cup fresh sliced fruit
　　1/2 grapefruit

3/4 cup fruit juice
1 medium-size orange, pear, banana, or apple

Dairy Products
1 cup milk or yogurt
1 slice cheese (American type)
1 one-inch cube other cheese

Note. Serving sizes: 3 teaspoons (tsp) = 1 tablespoon (tbsp) = 1/2 oz; using your
hand: 1 thumb size = 1 oz cheese; 1 palmful = 3 oz; 1 fist = 1 cup

Recently the USDA and the Food and Drug Administration (FDA)
required food companies to standardize their labels on packaged food.
Following is an explanation of these facts on the labels.

Serving Size: Sizes are standardized for the same types of food so
that they can be compared easily. Packaging also tells how many
serving sizes each package contains.

Amount Per Serving: Lists amounts of and calories from fat, carbohydrates, and protein. Also lists quantities of sodium, potassium, and vitamins.

Percent of Daily Value: Lists percent of calories supplied for a
daily intake of 2,000 or 2,500 calories. For example, if the food
provides 20 percent of the daily intake for fat, it gives you 400
calories from fat (2000 · .2 = 400). However, if you are on a
1,400-calorie diet, it will provide you 28.6 percent of calories
from fat (400 ÷ 1,400 = .286 = 28.6%), which is too much, of
course, for one food item.

Warning: Some foods will have a statement such as "No preservatives or artificial flavorings." Do not be misled by this statement.
Look for all additives, especially sulfites, bicarbonates, salicylates,
and artificial colors (e.g., tartrazine, which is in yellow and orange
colors). Some foods (e.g., hot sauces) do not have a food label.
Check the ingredients and don't be surprised to find some artificial
colors, which can cause serious allergies in some individuals.

RDAs Demystified

The Food and Nutrition Board first established Recommended Dietary Allowances (RDAs) in 1943 and has reviewed them every five
years since then. RDAs consider the absorption levels and metabolism rates of each nutrient averaged across age and sex categories for
the U.S. population.

In 1970, the Food and Drug Administration (FDA) started food labeling to inform consumers of the percentage of a nutrient's daily recommended requirement supplied by a particular food. The FDA chose the highest levels recommended by RDAs in 1968, concluding that by supplying the maximum daily levels, minimum needs would be met.

In 1992, the FDA suggested a new system using Reference Daily Intakes (RDIs), which would show the vitamin contents of foods by taking daily averages across age and sex groups, thus significantly decreasing the values listed on labels. More recent labels print a percent of daily value (% DV) that shows how much of the RDA a serving supplies, based on a daily caloric intake of 2,000 or 2,500 calories. Until food labeling is standardized and made easy for everyone to understand, the best way to evaluate food labels is to compare their contents with RDAs (see page 183 in Appendix B).

The Food and Nutrition Board has recently introduced new terminology that replaces RDAs. Although it will take a while for the new terminology and dietary intakes to be in general use, it is worthwhile to describe them now. RDAs have been replaced by Dietary Reference Intakes (DRI). DRIs are more complicated, but more accurately and scientifically represent the four values that follow.

- **Estimated Average Requirement (EAR):** The intake of a nutrient adequate to meet the requirement of half the healthy population.

- **Recommended Dietary Allowance (RDA):** Intake sufficient to meet the requirement of nearly all healthy persons in particular life-stage, age, and gender groups.

- **Adequate Intake (AI):** Intake estimates by groups of healthy people. They are used when reliable evidence is insufficient to determine an EAR and RDA value.

- **Tolerable Upper Intake Level (UL):** The highest level of intake likely to pose no risks of adverse health effects to most of the population.

The DRI table is available on page 185 of Appendix B.

Basic Foods and Their Functions

The major classes of nutrients are water, carbohydrates, fats, proteins, vitamins, and minerals. Each has an important place in our food plan,

PROPER HANDLING AND COOKING OF FOOD

Healthy eating is not possible without properly handling and cooking food. Many of the recent outbreaks related to contaminated food have resulted in unexpected fatalities. The following guidelines will help you to prepare, cook, and store foods properly.

- Wash your hands carefully and clean working surfaces (with bleach) when you are handling meat.
- Wash poultry thoroughly, inside and out.
- Cook meat thoroughly. Do not eat meat, especially seafood, raw.
- Frying, baking, and roasting foods for a long time will destroy nutrients, increase fat content, and produce carcinogens. That brown, tasty crust we all like on overcooked food contains carcinogenic compounds called nitrosamines. Thoroughly cooking foods for shorter periods under high temperatures by microwaving, steaming, or stir-frying will save their nutrients.
- Vegetables and fruits start losing their nutrients as soon as they are harvested. Furthermore, wilted and bruised vegetables are known to contain carcinogenic chemicals. Therefore, buy and eat fresh vegetables whenever possible. Frozen vegetables are a better choice than wilted or "stored fresh" vegetables as they retain more nutrients.
- Do not drown vegetables and fruits with water when you wash or cook them, since nutrients dissolve in water. Nevertheless, some of nutrients will always be lost to the cooking water. Do not throw away water left over from cooking but save it to use in preparing other dishes (e.g., soups, salads). Cook vegetables with as little water as possible and boil the water before you throw them in the pot. Keep the pot lid closed. These measures will shorten the cooking time, thus saving a lot of their nutrients as well as their color and flavor. Do not overcook them until they lose their natural color and crispiness.
- Some vegetables (e.g., onions, garlic, cabbage, cauliflower, broccoli, brussels sprouts, turnips, radishes) contain sulfur compounds. They should be boiled without a lid to get rid of the unpleasant odor and flavor.
- Refrigerate all foods immediately.
- Do not leave dirty dishes and wet sponges/washcloths for long periods (a couple of hours) as they are ideal places for bacteria to grow.
- Buy only pasteurized dairy products.

and overall health status is dependent on the proper amounts and mix of these nutrients.

Water

Water is generally ignored as a special nutrient, yet even a few days without water (leading to a loss of 9 to 12 percent of your body weight) is dangerous and can lead to death since 60 to 70 percent of your body weight is water. This is not the case for other nutrients, which we can survive without for considerable periods of time. Water is obtained from solid foods as well as from beverages. Some vegetables, such as potatoes, peas, and lettuce, are 75 to 96 percent water by weight.

Water must be replaced as it is lost during exercise to allow for sweat production. Failure to do so increases the chances of dehydration and eventually heat injury.

The amount of water stored in the body varies with one's diet. Carbohydrates require water for storage in the body. For example, 2.7 pounds of water is needed to store a pound of carbohydrate in the liver and muscles. When you begin a low-carbohydrate diet, the body's carbohydrate store decreases quickly over the next day or two, and the water stored with the carbohydrate is also lost. This helps to explain why you experience a rapid loss of body weight when you first begin such a diet. Keep in mind that you must have a negative balance of 3,500 calories to lose one pound of adipose (fat) tissue, a goal that virtually no one can achieve in one day.

Water is also very important in activating our fiber intake. The recommended 20 to 35 grams of daily fiber requires about six to eight glasses of water to be effective. Your daily water intake depends on the amount of calories you expend. You need about one milliliter of water (1 ml = 1 cc = 1/1000 L = 1/30 oz; 1 glass = 8 oz = 240 ml) for every calorie you burn. You lose water through sweat (24 oz), urine, feces, and breath air (12 oz) daily even when you are inactive.

Carbohydrates

Carbohydrates are a primary source of immediate energy in the diet, containing about four calories per gram. In the average American diet they make up only 45 percent of the calories, although the goal is 55 to 60 percent. Carbohydrates include foods that are digestible and can be used for energy (e.g., starches and sugars) and those that contain indigestible fiber. Sugars are found in jams, soft drinks, and milk, while starches are found in cereals, breads, and vegetables.

Fiber is an important component of the unprocessed (unrefined) carbohydrates we consume. Water-insoluble fiber found in leafy vegetables; roots; beans; unpeeled fruits; and whole grains such as oats, barley, rice, corn, and wheat (with sufficient water) forms bulk, softens stools, and keeps intestinal contents moving. It also slows absorption of sugars, carcinogens, and bile acids, which enhance the absorption of fats. Water-soluble fiber found in fruits, grains, seeds, and vegetables binds to bile acids and decreases the absorption of cholesterol.

Foods containing the highest fiber are kidney beans (9.3 grams per 3/4 cup), all-bran cereal (8.5 grams per 1/3 cup), and dried prunes (1.6 grams per prune). A daily intake of 10 to 13 grams of fiber per 1,000 calories is recommended. If your diet is not rich in fiber, you should increase your intake gradually to prevent gastrointestinal upsets. With sufficient fiber in your diet, your stools will float in the toilet bowl.

The following changes in diet are recommended to achieve the dietary goal of a reduction in refined and processed sugars and an increase in starches (complex carbohydrates) and fiber.

- Decrease consumption of soft drinks, cakes, cookies, and other foods containing sugar.
- Increase intake of whole-grain breads; cereals; fruits; and vegetables, including beans, lentils, and peas.

Rapid weight-loss diets simply cause a loss of body water that must, and eventually will, be replaced. Remember, it is the size of the negative caloric balance that is important in weight loss, not the type of diet. Given the dietary goals described previously, carbohydrates are the last food you should decrease in your diet when you plan to reduce body fat. Rapid weight-loss diets are usually very low in calories, lower than basal metabolic requirements. These diets cause an automatic reduction of metabolism to conserve energy, which in turn significantly decreases caloric expenditure. As a result, weight loss declines. We recommend that you compensate for an increase in complex carbohydrates, and therefore caloric intake, with a decrease in fat intake.

Fats

Fats are a primary source of energy, containing more than twice as many calories per gram (9 calories) as carbohydrates. Our main concern with fat is the structure of fatty acids it contains. Following is a brief description of fatty acids.

CHOOSING HEALTHY SNACKS

Many snacks, often those heavily advertised, contain simple processed sugars, saturated fats, and minimal fiber. The following guidelines will help you choose healthy snacks.

Change from the following unhealthy snacks:
Chocolate and candy bars
Cookies, cakes, and other pastry
Pretzels, corn and potato chips
Ice cream and whole milk
Fried vegetables, french fries

to the following healthy snacks:
Cocoa, prunes, raisins, apricots
Crackers and whole-grain muffins
Popcorn (no butter or salt), cereals (whole grain), nuts (with shell)
Skim milk, sherbet, yogurt
Fresh vegetables

Note. Avoid snacking on fast foods such as hamburgers, hot dogs, french fries, and pizza, which are loaded with saturated fats.

• Foods containing saturated fatty acids contain cholesterol, are solid at room temperature, and generally are derived from animal foods. Exceptions are coconut oil and palm oil. Saturated fatty acids raise both LDL-C and HDL-C.

• Foods containing monounsaturated fatty acids (MUSFA, one double bond) and polyunsaturated fatty acids (PUSFA, more than one double bond) are lower in cholesterol, are liquid at room temperature, and in general are derived from plant foods (e.g., olive oil, a MUSFA). Linoleic acid, also known as N-6 fatty acid, is a PUSFA and belongs to a class of essential fatty acids that are mainly derived from cold-water fish (e.g., salmon, black cod, tuna), milk, and breast milk. Corn, sunflower, peanut, and soybean oils also contain PUSFA. PUSFA lowers LDL-C and causes no change in HDL-C. MUSFA lowers LDL-C and increases HDL-C.

Eskimos rarely suffer from heart disease or stroke despite their high-fat diet. The major source of fat in their diet is fish. Fish, one of the leanest sources of protein, provides polyunsaturated fat, which is structurally quite different from the fat we eat with red meat or chicken.

- N-3 fatty acids are derived from plant and seafood sources. Plant sources provide a medium-chain fatty acid. Seafood provides long-chain fatty acids. Plant sources of N-3 fatty acids have been shown to protect against coronary artery disease more than seafood sources. These fatty acids lower LDL-C and raise HDL-C.

- Vegetable oils become hardened with partial hydrogenation, forming *trans fatty acids*, a major fat component of commercially cooked foods such as french fries, cookies, crackers, and margarine. Trans fatty acids raise LDL-C and lower HDL-C and are known as the foods most detrimental to heart and blood vessels.

Note. Recent studies have shown that one's intake of saturated and trans fatty acids can be reduced by half by eliminating butter, margarine, dairy products containing 2 percent fat or whole milk, and meats with fat.

Although there is no difference in the number of calories per gram for liquid or solid fats, there are major differences between the two in terms of good health. The consumption of large amounts of saturated dietary fats is associated with higher rates of heart disease. It should be no surprise, then, that the recommended dietary goals (see table 4.1) include a reduction in total fat consumption to 30 percent or less and an additional cutback in saturated fats to 5–10 percent. This is also true for cholesterol (another type of fat), for which a dietary goal of less than 300 milligrams per day has been established.

To accomplish these goals, the following guidelines are recommended:

- Eat more lean meat, fish, poultry, and dry beans and peas as sources of protein.
- Use skim or low-fat milk and milk products.
- Limit your consumption of eggs and organ meats.
- Limit your intake of fats and oils, especially those high in saturated fats, such as butter, lard, shortening, and foods containing palm and coconut oils.
- Broil, bake, or boil rather than fry, and trim fat off meat.

Protein

Protein, like carbohydrates, provides four calories per gram; protein, however, is not viewed as a primary energy source. Protein is an important nutrient because it contains amino acids necessary for tissue growth, development, and repair. High-quality protein is found in eggs, meat, fish, milk, poultry, cheese, and soybeans. Grains, vegetables, seeds, and nuts provide lower-quality protein; more of this is required per day than the higher-quality protein.

The protein requirement for an adult is only 0.8 gram per kilogram of body weight, so a 154-pound (70-kilogram) person needs only 56 grams, or about two ounces, per day. A rapidly growing baby requires 2.2 grams per kilogram of body weight. About 12 percent of the average American's food intake is protein, which is sufficient to meet this standard.

Vitamins

Vitamins are special nutrients required in very small amounts but vital for normal function. They are classified as *fat soluble* or *water soluble* based on their ability to dissolve in lipids or in water. Fat-soluble vitamins include A, D, E, and K. Because of their solubility, they can be stored in the body and are not needed every day since you can "catch up" on other days.

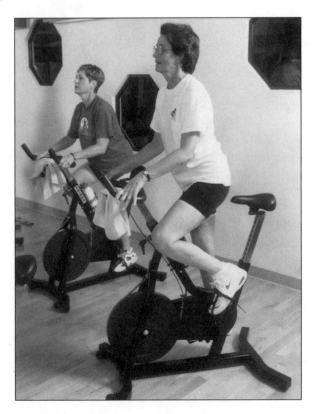

Fat-soluble vitamins are stored in body fat. A potential problem with them is that if too much is taken in over a long period of time, they can cause hypervitaminosis, a toxicity condition that can lead to nervous disorders, gastrointestinal problems, and damage to your liver and kidneys.

Water-soluble vitamins, which include the B vitamins, C, folic acid, pantothenic acid, and biotin, are much less likely to induce hypervitaminosis, since any excess is excreted in the urine. However, high levels of water-soluble vitamins can also be toxic and should be avoided. Due to the high turnover of water-soluble vitamins, you need to replace your supplies on a daily basis.

A summary of these vitamins, their functions, and their food sources is presented in table 4.3. The last two columns of the table list the adult requirements for each vitamin. These values are taken from the tables of Recommended Dietary Allowances (RDA) and Estimated Safe and Adequate Daily Dietary Intakes found in appendix B and are consistent with the requirements of healthy people. Requirements are different for men, children, women, and pregnant or breast-feeding women. Although these are the values you can use to evaluate the adequacy of your diet, do not expect to meet each requirement on a daily basis. Evaluate your diet over a period of several days to see if your intake is adequate on the average.

Should you take a vitamin supplement? If you are eating a varied diet containing the major food groups (discussion follows), you do not need a vitamin supplement. If you want to make sure you're getting all the vitamins, taking a single multivitamin every other day will generally not cause problems. However, commonly advertised and consumed vitamin supplements that exceed RDAs or the "megavitamins" can lead to hypervitaminosis, a serious health problem. Following is a list of vitamins and the results of taking them in excess.

- Vitamin A—blindness and fetus abnormalities
- Vitamin C—kidney stones and the destruction of B_{12} in food
- Vitamin D—kidney stones
- Vitamin E—interference with the function of vitamin K
- Niacin—liver injury

It is better to focus your attention on eating a balanced diet to meet these vitamin needs in the long run than to depend on a supplement. Remember, by eating a balanced diet, you also fulfill protein and mineral requirements.

Table 4.3

Vitamins and Their Functions

Vitamin	Function	Sources	DAILY ADULT REQUIREMENT[a]	
			Men	Women
Thiamin (B₁)	Functions as part of a coenzyme to aid energy use	Whole grains, nuts, lean pork	1.5 mg	1.1 mg
Riboflavin (B₂)	Involved in energy metabolism as part of a coenzyme	Milk, yogurt, cheese	1.7 mg	1.3 mg
Niacin	Facilitates energy production in cells	Lean meat, fish, poultry, grains	19.0 mg	15.0 mg
B₆	Absorbs and metabolizes protein; aids in red blood cell formation	Lean meat, vegetables, whole grains	2.0 mg	1.6 mg
Pantothenic acid	Aids in metabolism of carbohydrate, fat, and protein	Whole-grain cereals, bread, dark green vegetables	4–7 mg	4–7 mg
Folate	Functions as coenzyme in synthesis of nucleic acids and protein	Green vegetables, beans, whole-wheat products	200 μg	180 μg
B₁₂	Involved in synthesis of nucleic acids, red blood cell formation	Only in animal foods, not plant foods	2 μg	2 μg
Biotin	Coenzyme in synthesis of fatty acids and glycogen formation	Egg yolk, dark green vegetables	20–30 μg	20–30 μg
C	Intracellular maintenance of bone, capillaries, and teeth	Citrus fruits, green peppers, tomatoes	60 mg	60 mg
A	Functions in visual processes; formation and maintenance of skin and mucous membranes	Carrots, sweet potatoes, margarine, butter, liver	1,000 μg RE	800 μg RE
D	Aids in growth and formation of bones and teeth; promotes calcium absorption	Eggs, tuna, liver, fortified milk	5 mg[b]	5 mg[b]
E	Protects polyunsaturated fats; prevents cell membrane damage	Vegetable oils, whole-grain cereal and bread, green leafy vegetables	10 mg	8 mg
K	Important in blood clotting	Green leafy vegetables, peas, potatoes	80 μg	65 μg

mg = milligram; μg = microgram; RE = retinol equivalent
[a]Values are for adults 25 to 50 years of age. Values are from National Research Council (1989), *Recommended Dietary Allowances*, 10th ed. The requirements vary for children and pregnant or lactating women.
[b]For adults over 50 years of age, increase to 10–15 milligrams per day.

Reprinted, by permission, from E.T. Howley and B.D. Franks, 1986, *Health Fitness Instructor's Handbook.* (Champaign, IL: Human Kinetics), 65.

Minerals

Minerals are chemical elements that, like vitamins, are needed in small amounts for normal health. They are divided into two classes: *major minerals* and *trace minerals*. Major minerals include calcium, which is needed for bones; potassium and sodium, which are needed for nerve and muscle function; and magnesium, which is needed for many of the body's enzymes to function. Potassium and calcium also play an important role in the function of the heart muscle. Trace minerals include iron, which is needed by hemoglobin to transport oxygen in the red blood cells; iodine, which is necessary for the hormone thyroxine, needed to keep our metabolic rates at the right level; and zinc, selenium, copper, and others, which are needed for certain enzymes to function properly.

You can achieve the daily requirements for most of these minerals by eating a varied and balanced diet. However, there is some concern that women do not take in sufficient amounts of iron and calcium; women may opt for supplementation of these minerals. Table 4.4 presents a summary of the major and trace minerals, their food sources, and adult requirements.

Table salt is sodium chloride, 40 percent of which is sodium. A teaspoon of salt contains about 2.3 grams (2,300 milligrams) of sodium. Since adults only need 220 milligrams of sodium, it is best to keep our sodium intake as low as possible. One should keep in mind that *all foods contain sodium. Thus, we take in sufficient sodium even if salt is not added to our food before or after cooking.* Condiments and salad dressings contain huge amounts of sodium per teaspoonful: baking soda contains 821 milligrams; meat tenderizer contains 1,750 milligrams; one dill pickle contains 928 milligrams; and soy sauce contains 1,029 milligrams. Among natural foods (per serving), milk (126 mg), yogurt (105 mg), meat (65 mg), raw carrots (25 mg), spinach (22 mg), and cornmeal (43 mg) are rich sources of sodium. These natural foods also provide other important minerals such as potassium and magnesium. The following guidelines are recommended to reduce salt intake:

- Use minimal salt in cooking.
- Add herbs and spices instead of salt to food.
- Cut back on canned, frozen, and processed foods. Even low-calorie diet dinners contain large amounts of sodium. Before buying these foods, read their labels for sodium content.

Table 4.4

Minerals and Their Functions

Mineral	Function	Sources	DAILY ADULT REQUIREMENT[a] Men	Women
		Major minerals		
Calcium	Bones, teeth, blood clotting, nerve and muscle function	Milk, sardines, dark green vegetables, nuts	1,200 mg	1,200 mg[b]
Chloride	Nerve and muscle function, water balance (with sodium)	Table salt	750 mg	750 mg
Magnesium	Bone growth; nerve, muscle, and enzyme function	Nuts, seafood, whole grains, leafy green vegetables	350 mg	280 mg
Phosphorus	Bone, teeth, energy transfer	Meats, poultry, seafood, eggs, milk, beans	800 mg	800 mg
Potassium	Nerve and muscle function	Fresh vegetables, bananas, citrus fruits, milk, meats, fish	2,000 mg	2,000 mg
Sodium	Nerve and muscle function, water balance	Table salt	500 mg	500 mg
		Trace minerals		
Chromium	Glucose metabolism	Meats, liver, whole grains, dried beans	.05–.2 mg	.05–.2 mg
Copper	Enzyme function, energy production	Meats, seafood, nuts, grains	1.5–3 mg	1.5–3 mg
Fluoride	Bone and teeth growth	Drinking water, fish, milk	1.5–4 mg	1.5–4 mg
Iodine	Thyroid hormone formation	Iodized salt, seafood	150 μg	150 μg
Iron	O_2 transport in red blood cells; enzyme function	Red meat, liver, eggs, beans, leafy vegetables, shellfish	10 mg	15 mg
Manganese	Enzyme function	Whole grains, nuts, fruits, vegetables	2.5–5 mg	2.5–5 mg
Molybdenum	Energy metabolism in cells	Whole grains, organ meats, peas, beans	75–250 mg	75–250 mg
Selenium	Works with vitamin E	Meat, fish, whole grains, eggs	70 μg	55 μg
Zinc	Part of enzymes; growth	Meat, shellfish, yeast, whole grains	15 mg	12 mg

[a]Values are for adults 23 to 50 years of age. The requirements vary for children and pregnant or lactating women.
[b]For postmenopausal women, increase to 1,500 milligrams per day.
Based on data from J.L. Christian and J.L. Greger (1985) and M.H. Williams (1988).

Antioxidants and Prevention

Our bodies naturally produce "free radicals," which damage cells by oxidation, enhance aging, and promote cancer development. The body's natural defense against these chemicals is limited by exposure to cigarette smoke, air pollution, radiation, sunlight, and stress. Oxidation also plays an important role in the buildup of cholesterol in arteries. Many studies have shown that antioxidants found in vitamins A (beta carotene), C, and E and minerals such as selenium; flavonoids in citrus fruits; sulfides in garlic and onions; isothiocyanates in cabbage, broccoli, and cauliflower; and phenolic compounds in tea prevent the development of cancers. Isoflavones in soy products and lignin in whole wheat suppress estrogen levels, which play an important role in the development of breast cancer.

Evaluating Your Dietary Intake

How do you know whether you are taking in the number of calories needed to maintain or lose weight? The first step is to complete a dietary record that will give you a sense of how food fits into your life. Answer the following questions:

- How many times a day do you eat?
- Do you enjoy eating?
- Do you eat when you are hungry or according to a time schedule?
- When do you eat meals?
- When do you eat snacks?
- What foods do you eat most often?
- What are your favorite snacks?
- What are some of your least favorite foods?
- How long does it take you to eat a meal?
- Do you eat more or less than other people?
- Are you on a diet? What kind?
- Do you use vitamin and mineral supplements?

Socialize by cooking for your family and friends instead of eating out on special occasions.

- How much solid fat (butter, margarine, lard) do you use?
- Do you add salt to your food while cooking?
- Do you use low-fat or regular dairy products?
- How many times a week do you eat meat, poultry, and fish, and what size portions do you eat?
- Do you primarily fry, bake, broil, or boil your meat?
- How often do you eat vegetables and fruits?
- How long has your weight been what it is now?
- When you eat at home, who does the cooking?
- How often do you eat out?

This review gives you an idea of how your dietary habits compare to the recommendations mentioned earlier regarding reducing fat intake and increasing consumption of complex carbohydrates. Further, by focusing attention on how you cook food, when and where you eat, your likes and dislikes, and your favorite snacks, you can begin to control your caloric intake.

If you always find yourself eating snacks in your easy chair while watching television, there may be an association between eating the snack and the comfort of the TV room. Changing any habits, including dietary ones, may first require you to change the circumstances associated with the habits. If you restrict all your eating to the kitchen, you may find your eating habits easier to change. An additional discussion on how to change habits is presented in chapter 2.

EATING HABITS

Our eating habits and daily activities significantly influence each other. The following guidelines will help to coordinate these activities and decrease negative influences.

- Intense exercise before meals may blunt appetite and prevent gorging. It reduces the ready source of energy called glycogen and aids the storage of carbohydrates taken with the meal. Intense exercise after meals disrupts digestion by shunting blood away from the digestive tract to muscles. However, mild exercise after meals (e.g., walking) helps digestion, increases caloric expenditure, and controls weight gain.

Therefore, lying down after meals or snacking at bedtime will not help digestion but will result in more of the food energy being stored.

- Intense exercise, heavy and spicy meals, caffeine, and excess alcohol and tobacco use before bedtime will keep you from sleeping well.

- Relax while you are eating and eat slowly. Do not engage in active conversation while you have food in your mouth. Chew your food well to enjoy it and to mix it with your saliva since digestion starts in the mouth.

- Brush your teeth after each meal. If this does not seem feasible after lunch, as is true for many of us, then rinse your mouth well.

- Establish a regular schedule for meals, exercise, and rest so that your body can efficiently handle each activity. The gastrointestinal system, although very vulnerable to mood, is very prone to conditioning. A little physical activity, 10 to 15 minutes every morning, will stimulate your metabolism and circulation, and then sitting on the toilet for five minutes will provide you regular bowel movements.

- Do not eat others' leftovers and do not drink from others' glasses.

- Our skin is always contaminated with pathogens (e.g., staphylococcus). These bacteria grow very fast in food. Therefore, wash your hands before and after eating.

- To prevent exercise-related GI problems, follow these guidelines before exercising:
  1. Decrease fiber intake.
  2. Drink plenty of water or low-sugar drinks (less than 10 percent).
  3. Do not take anti-inflammatory medicines, including steroids.
  4. Eat foods low in fat and protein (both take longer to digest) and rich in carbohydrates.
  5. Do not eat very spicy and gas-producing foods (e.g., beans, broccoli, cabbage).
  6. Wait two to three hours after you eat before exercising vigorously.

What to Avoid

There is no question about the interest in the topics of health and weight control—just look at all the dietary books and programs for sale in every community. Unfortunately, but not surprisingly, some books and programs provide incorrect and potentially dangerous information regarding diet, exercise, and weight loss. The purpose of this section is to discuss some of the fads and gimmicks that are sold under the pretense that they will help a person achieve a weight-loss goal.

Most people who lose weight regain it within a year because they have not dealt with the factors involved in the energy balance equation: energy expenditure and caloric intake. In addition, they have not paid attention to changing the lifestyle behaviors related to their patterns of eating and exercise. Authorities generally recommend that you create a caloric imbalance of about 500 to 1,000 calories per day through modifications in diet and exercise. This adjustment will cause the loss of about one or two pounds per week and allow you to gain control over exercise and eating behaviors.

We cannot overemphasize the need to make small and systematic changes in your diet and activity levels to achieve and maintain your target weight. In the process you will learn how to plan meals better to meet your dietary goals and RDA standards. We have provided a checklist (table 4.5) to help you make decisions about weight-loss diets; the next time you are considering a diet, use the checklist to help you.

There is no lack of fad diets and commercial enterprises that promise an incredible weight loss in a short period of time. As we mentioned earlier, there is money to be made, and you need to be wary of exaggerated claims. The saying "If it's too good to be true, it probably is" is a good one to remember when you are considering diets and gimmicks. We would like to comment on a few of the more common gimmicks used to "lose" weight.

• *Diuretics.* These drugs cause sodium, potassium, and water loss from the body. The weight change that occurs as a result is therefore unrelated to body fatness.

• *Laxatives.* These medications are usually used to loosen fecal matter in the large intestine and promote bowel movements. People who use laxatives for weight loss are under the illusion that if laxatives speed things along the intestinal tract, some food will not be absorbed into the body. This is not true. Laxatives have little effect on absorption but instead cause the loss of important minerals and water from the body.

• *"Sauna" suits.* These suits are made of materials impermeable to sweat, which must be evaporated from the surface of the skin to cool

Table 4.5

Weight-Loss Diet Evaluation Checklist

The following checklist can be used to evaluate weight-loss diets. A *No* answer to any of the questions indicates an inadequate weight-reduction plan. Does your diet

	Yes	No
1. Aim for a weight loss of one to two pounds per week?	☐	☐
2. Provide at least 1,200 calories per day?	☐	☐
3. Recommend a regular endurance exercise program?	☐	☐
4. Provide a balance of foods from all four food groups?	☐	☐
5. Provide for variety to prevent boredom?	☐	☐
6. Establish eating and exercise habits that can be maintained the rest of your life?	☐	☐
7. Conform to your personal lifestyle?	☐	☐
8. Work without pills, drugs, or other gadgets?	☐	☐

Reprinted, by permission, from E.T. Howley and B.D. Franks, 1986, *Health Fitness Instructor's Handbook*. (Champaign, IL: Human Kinetics), 73.

the body during exercise. Because evaporation does not occur when these suits are worn, the body sweats more in an attempt to cool itself. This results in a loss of water weight that will (and must) be replaced as soon as possible. These suits do not "burn" calories away. Sitting in a sauna has the same effect on water weight.

• *Elastic belts.* These belts are worn around the waist and allegedly "melt" fat away, causing changes in your waist size. Your waist size does decrease as tissues are compressed; within a few hours, however, the tissues return to their normal size and the effect disappears.

• *Vibrators or massagers.* These devices promise to break up fat in localized areas, cause "spot reduction," and speed weight loss. "Spot reduction" is a dream that can't come true because weight is lost from the body in a pattern opposite to the way it went on. If the fat went to your hips first and your face last, it will come from your face first and your hips last when you lose body fat. These machines may be enjoyable to use, but they do not increase energy expenditure, which is the necessary ingredient in weight loss.

• *Appetite suppressants/diet pills.* These medicines are indicated only for people with serious medical problems related to obesity. They work only with an effective low-calorie diet and exercise program. People who rely only on these pills for losing weight regain their weight and usually more when they stop taking them. Excess weight develops over a period of years. Therefore, to expect to lose it in a short time is not only unrealistic but also very dangerous to health. The majority of these drugs can increase blood pressure and heart rate and cause irregular heartbeats. Depression, drowsiness, abdominal pain, major sleep problems, jitteriness, and headaches are not uncommon with their use. Some of these medicines have been withdrawn from the market because of their serious side effects such as heart valve problems and fatal pulmonary hypertension. Furthermore, some of these pills will result in positive drug screens, while others are scheduled as controlled drugs because of their potential for addiction.

We hope that you now have a better understanding of food, your relationship to it, and the fundamentals of healthy eating. By objectively examining your eating habits and diet and making educated and sensible changes that you can adhere to over the long haul, you are on your way to improving your health and fitness.

chapter **5**

Aerobic Fitness

Aerobic fitness is a good measure of your heart's ability to pump oxygen-rich blood to the muscles. Exercise scientists call aerobic fitness "maximal oxygen uptake" and abbreviate it as $\dot{V}O_2$max. It is also called cardiovascular or cardiorespiratory fitness (CRF). Although there are technical differences among the terms *cardio* (heart), *vascular* (blood vessels), *respiratory* (lungs), and *aerobic* (working with oxygen), they all reflect various aspects of this component of fitness. We will use these terms in a general way to represent this fitness area. A person with a healthy, large heart can pump great volumes of blood with each beat and has a high level of CRF.

Measures of Aerobic Fitness

Cardiorespiratory fitness values are expressed in the following ways: the number of liters of oxygen used by the body per minute (L/min), the number of milliliters of oxygen used per kilogram of body weight per minute (ml/kg/min), and METs. One MET describes the amount of oxygen used by the body at rest and is equal to 3.5 ml/kg/min. If you use 35 ml/kg/min during maximal exercise, you are said to have a CRF equal to 10 METs ($35 \div 3.5 = 10$).

Because aerobic training programs increase the heart's ability to pump blood, they result in increased CRF. Most tests used to evaluate CRF use dynamic activities, those involving the large muscle groups in the legs (usually walking, running, stepping, or cycling). The following sections suggest how to approach such tests, what information they offer, and how to interpret them.

Sequence for Testing and Activities

The guidelines presented in chapter 1 will help you decide when to take fitness tests and participate in fitness activities. Generally, the testing process begins with a series of resting measurements, which may include a blood sample, a heart rate measure, a blood pressure measure, an electrocardiogram (ECG), pulmonary measures to evaluate lung function, and of course, a body fatness measure. The number and types of measurements will depend on your age, apparent health status, and your fitness program facility (if any). Clearly, if you are exercising on your own, you are less likely to obtain sophisticated measurements prior to the fitness tests. If you have known medical problems or are at high risk, you should have a physical examination prior to taking a fitness test or starting an exercise program.

If the resting measurements indicate that you can take a fitness test, we recommend a *submaximal* fitness test. Submaximal tests *do not* require you to exercise to your maximum effort, and they reduce the chance that you will have sore muscles the next day. Heart rate and blood pressure are usually measured, and the test is stopped at 70 to 85 percent of estimated maximal heart rate. The results provide useful information related to your CRF, and the test is a sensitive indicator of how you improve over time. In some testing centers an ECG is also obtained, depending on the person being tested and the personnel involved. If your measurements are normal, you are ready to start a fitness program; if not, you may be referred for additional tests or procedures.

In some testing centers the submaximal test is continued past this point, and you may be asked to exercise to maximum. This is more likely in a clinical setting, where using this kind of maximal test increases the chance of finding any abnormalities. However, some maximal tests only measure the time it takes to run a given distance. This type of maximal test is *not recommended* at the start of a fitness program because it requires an all-out effort and blood pressure and ECG are not monitored.

Field Tests

A variety of tests can be used to obtain an estimate of CRF. They are called "field tests" because they require very little equipment, can be done just about anywhere, and use the simple activities of walking and running. Because these tests require you to walk or run as fast as you can over a set distance, they are not recommended at the start of an exercise program. Instead, we recommend that you begin with the graduated walking and/or jogging programs outlined in chapter 10 before taking these tests. A graduated fitness program will allow you to start at a low, safe level of activity and gradually improve. After you become physically active it is appropriate for you to take a test to see how fit you are.

Because the heart must pump great volumes of oxygen to the muscles when you walk or run at high speeds over long distances, the average speed you maintain in these field tests gives an estimate of your CRF. The higher your CRF score, the greater the capacity of the heart to transport oxygen.

Walk Test

The one-mile walk test was developed as a CRF test for adults, especially older adults. The test should be done on a measured track or other flat surface so that the distance of one mile is clearly identified. For example, four laps on an outdoor running track is usually equal to one mile. If you use an indoor track, mall, or gymnasium, check with someone to make sure of the distance.

Do the test in the cooler part of the day and stretch out and do some slow walking to warm up. The idea for the test is simply to walk the mile as fast as you can (do not run or jog). Use a stopwatch to record your time in minutes and seconds. In addition, at the end of the walk, stop and *immediately* take your heart rate for 10 seconds. (If you use a "heart watch" to check your heart rate during exercise, record your heart rate for the last half-lap.)

Knowing the time it took you to walk the mile and your heart rate value, you can use table 5.1 to estimate your CRF (data used to generate the table are from Kline et al., 1987). Find the section of the table pertaining to your sex and age, then read across the top until you find the time (to the nearest minute) it took you to walk the mile. Look down that column until it intersects with your heart rate (listed in the far left column). That number is your CRF value in terms of oxygen used per kilogram of body weight per minute.

You can evaluate your aerobic fitness by comparing the number you obtained from table 5.1 with the standards presented in table 5.2. For example, a 25-year-old man who walks the mile in 20 minutes and has a heart rate of 140 has an estimated maximal oxygen uptake of 29.2 ml/kg/min. Based on table 5.2, his maximal oxygen uptake is "borderline," indicating the need for improvement.

Jog/Run Test

One of the most common CRF field tests is the 12-minute or 1.5-mile run popularized by Dr. Kenneth Cooper. This test is very much like the walk test just described: participants jog or run as fast as they can for 12 minutes or for 1.5 miles. Since your average running speed is dependent on the ability of your heart and lungs to transport oxygen to the working muscles, your CRF score is based on the speed you can maintain over the distance. Remember, this test is not to be done at the beginning of a fitness program; wait until you have progressed

Table 5.1

Estimated Maximal Oxygen Uptake (ml/kg/min) for Men and Women, 20-69 Years Old

HR	10	11	12	13	14	15	16	17	18	19	20
					MIN/MI						
					Men (20–29)						
120	65.0	61.7	58.4	55.2	51.9	48.6	45.4	42.1	38.9	35.6	32.3
130	63.4	60.1	56.9	53.6	50.3	47.1	43.8	40.6	37.3	34.0	30.8
140	61.8	58.6	55.3	52.0	48.8	45.5	42.2	39.0	35.7	32.5	29.2
150	60.3	57.0	53.7	50.5	47.2	43.9	40.7	37.4	34.2	30.9	27.6
160	58.7	55.4	52.2	48.9	45.6	42.4	39.1	35.9	32.6	29.3	26.1
170	57.1	53.9	50.6	47.3	44.1	40.8	37.6	34.3	31.0	27.8	24.5
180	55.6	52.3	49.0	45.8	42.5	39.3	36.0	32.7	29.5	26.2	22.9
190	54.0	50.7	47.5	44.2	41.0	37.7	34.4	31.2	27.9	24.6	21.4
200	52.4	49.2	45.9	42.7	39.4	36.1	32.9	29.6	26.3	23.1	19.8
					Women (20–29)						
120	62.1	58.9	55.6	52.3	49.1	45.8	42.5	39.3	36.0	32.7	29.5
130	60.6	57.3	54.0	50.8	47.5	44.2	41.0	37.7	34.4	31.2	27.9
140	59.0	55.7	52.5	49.2	45.9	42.7	39.4	36.1	32.9	29.6	26.3
150	57.4	54.2	50.9	47.6	44.4	41.1	37.8	34.6	31.3	28.0	24.8
160	55.9	52.6	49.3	46.7	42.8	39.5	36.3	33.0	29.7	26.5	23.2
170	54.3	51.0	47.8	44.5	41.2	38.0	34.7	31.4	28.2	24.9	21.6
180	52.7	49.5	46.2	42.9	39.7	36.4	33.1	29.9	26.6	23.3	20.1
190	51.2	47.9	44.6	41.4	38.1	34.8	31.6	28.3	25.0	21.8	18.5
200	49.6	46.3	43.1	39.8	36.5	33.3	30.0	26.7	23.5	20.2	16.9

(continued)

Table 5.1 (continued)

						MIN/MI					
HR	10	11	12	13	14	15	16	17	18	19	20
						Men (30–39)					
120	61.1	57.8	54.6	51.3	48.0	44.8	41.5	38.2	35.0	31.7	28.4
130	59.5	56.3	53.0	49.7	46.5	43.2	39.9	36.7	33.4	30.1	26.9
140	58.0	54.7	51.4	48.2	44.9	41.6	38.4	35.1	31.8	28.6	25.3
150	56.4	53.4	49.9	46.6	43.3	40.1	36.8	33.5	30.3	27.0	23.8
160	54.8	51.6	48.3	45.0	41.8	38.5	35.2	32.0	28.7	25.5	22.2
170	53.3	50.0	46.7	43.5	40.2	36.9	33.7	30.4	27.1	23.9	20.6
180	51.7	48.4	45.2	41.9	38.6	35.4	32.1	28.8	25.6	22.3	19.1
190	50.1	46.9	43.6	40.3	37.1	33.8	30.5	27.3	24.0	20.8	17.5
						Women (30–39)					
120	58.2	55.0	51.7	48.4	45.2	41.9	38.7	35.4	32.1	28.9	25.6
130	56.7	53.4	50.1	46.9	43.6	40.4	37.1	33.8	30.6	27.3	24.0
140	55.1	51.8	48.6	45.3	42.1	38.8	35.5	32.3	29.0	24.7	22.5
150	53.5	50.3	47.0	43.8	40.5	37.2	34.0	30.7	27.4	24.2	20.9
160	52.0	48.7	45.4	42.2	38.9	35.7	32.4	29.1	25.9	22.6	19.3
170	50.4	47.1	43.9	40.6	37.4	34.1	30.8	27.6	24.3	21.0	17.8
180	48.8	45.6	42.3	39.1	35.8	32.5	29.3	26.0	22.7	19.5	16.2
190	47.3	44.0	40.8	37.5	34.2	31.0	27.7	24.4	21.2	17.9	14.6

(continued)

Table 5.1 (continued)

						MIN/MI						
HR	10	11	12	13	14	15	16	17	18	19	20
Men (40–49)											
120	57.2	54.0	50.7	47.4	44.2	40.9	37.6	34.4	31.1	27.8	24.6
130	55.7	52.4	49.1	45.9	42.6	39.3	36.1	32.8	29.5	26.3	23.0
140	54.1	50.8	47.6	44.3	41.0	37.8	34.5	31.2	28.0	24.7	21.4
150	52.5	49.3	46.0	42.7	39.5	36.2	32.9	29.7	26.4	23.1	19.9
160	51.0	47.7	44.4	41.2	37.9	34.6	31.4	28.1	24.8	21.6	18.3
170	49.4	46.1	42.9	39.6	36.3	33.1	29.8	26.5	23.3	20.0	16.7
180	47.8	44.6	41.3	38.0	34.8	31.5	28.2	25.0	21.7	18.4	15.2
Women (40–49)											
120	54.4	51.1	47.8	44.6	41.3	38.0	34.8	31.5	28.2	25.0	21.7
130	52.8	49.5	46.3	43.0	39.7	36.5	33.2	29.9	26.7	23.4	20.1
140	51.2	48.0	44.7	41.4	38.2	34.9	31.6	28.4	25.1	21.8	18.6
150	49.7	46.4	43.1	39.9	36.6	33.3	30.1	26.8	23.5	20.3	17.0
160	48.1	44.8	41.6	38.3	35.0	31.8	28.5	25.2	22.0	18.7	15.5
170	46.5	43.3	40.0	36.7	33.5	30.2	26.9	23.7	20.4	17.2	13.9
Men (50–59)											
120	53.3	50.0	46.8	43.5	40.3	37.0	33.7	30.5	27.2	23.9	20.7
130	51.7	48.5	45.2	42.0	38.7	35.4	32.2	28.9	25.6	22.4	19.1
140	50.2	46.9	43.7	40.4	37.1	33.9	30.6	27.3	24.1	20.8	17.5
150	48.6	45.4	42.1	38.8	35.6	32.3	29.0	25.8	22.5	19.2	16.0
160	47.1	43.8	40.5	37.3	34.0	30.7	27.5	24.2	20.9	17.7	14.4
170	45.5	42.2	39.0	35.7	32.4	29.2	25.9	22.6	19.4	16.1	12.8

(continued)

Table 5.1 (continued)

HR	10	11	12	13	14	15	16	17	18	19	20
					Women (50–59)						
120	50.5	47.2	43.9	40.7	37.4	34.1	30.9	27.6	24.3	21.1	17.8
130	48.9	45.6	42.4	39.1	35.8	32.6	29.3	26.0	22.8	19.5	16.2
140	47.3	44.1	40.8	37.5	34.3	31.0	27.7	24.5	21.2	17.9	14.7
150	45.8	42.5	39.2	36.0	32.7	29.4	26.2	22.9	19.6	16.4	13.1
160	44.2	40.9	37.7	34.4	31.1	27.9	24.6	21.3	18.1	14.8	11.5
170	42.6	39.4	36.1	32.8	29.6	26.3	23.0	19.8	16.5	13.2	10.0
					Men (60–69)						
120	49.4	46.2	42.9	39.6	36.4	33.1	29.8	26.6	23.3	20.0	16.8
130	47.9	44.6	41.3	38.1	34.8	31.5	28.3	25.0	21.7	18.5	15.2
140	46.3	43.0	39.8	36.5	33.2	30.0	26.7	23.4	20.2	16.9	13.6
150	44.7	41.5	38.2	34.9	31.7	28.4	25.1	21.9	18.6	15.3	12.1
160	43.2	39.9	36.6	33.4	30.1	26.8	23.6	20.3	17.0	13.8	10.5
					Women (60–69)						
120	46.6	43.3	40.0	36.8	33.5	30.2	27.0	23.7	20.5	17.2	13.9
130	45.0	41.7	38.5	35.2	31.9	28.7	25.4	22.2	18.9	15.6	12.4
140	43.4	40.2	36.9	33.6	30.4	27.1	23.8	20.6	17.3	14.1	10.8
150	41.9	38.6	35.3	32.1	28.8	25.5	22.3	19.0	15.8	12.5	9.2
160	40.3	37.0	33.8	30.5	27.2	24.0	20.7	17.5	14.2	10.9	7.7

Note. Calculations assume 170 lb for men and 125 lb for women. For each 15 lb beyond these values, subtract 1 ml/kg/min.

Reprinted, by permission, from E.T. Howley and B.D. Franks, 1997, *Health Fitness Instructor's Handbook*, 3d ed. (Champaign, IL: Human Kinetics), 209–210.

to a jogging program. Find a measured track and run as far as you can in 12 minutes, or run 1.5 miles for time.

Table 5.2 lists values for CRF as "good," "adequate," "borderline," and "needs extra work," taking age and sex into consideration. For example, a 40-year-old woman who runs 1.5 miles in 14 minutes and 15 seconds (14:15) rates between "adequate" and "good." This time of 14:15 corresponds to a CRF value of about 35 to 40 ml/kg/min. We

Table 5.2
Standards for Maximal Oxygen Uptake and Endurance Runs

Age[a]	$\dot{V}O_2max$ (ml/kg/min)		1.5-mi run (min:s)		12-min run (mi)	
	Female[b]	Male	Female	Male	Female	Male
Good						
15–30	>40	>45	<12	<10	>1.5	>1.7
35–50	>35	>40	<13:30	<11:30	>1.4	>1.5
55–70	>30	>35	<16	<14	>1.2	>1.3
Adequate for most activities						
15–30	35	40	13:30	11:50	1.4	1.5
35–50	30	35	15	13	1.3	1.4
55–70	25	30	17:30	15:30	1.1	1.3
Borderline						
15–30	30	35	15	13	1.3	1.4
35–50	25	30	16:30	14:30	1.2	1.3
55–70	20	25	19	17	1.0	1.2
Needs extra work on CRF						
15–30	<25	<30	>17	>15	<1.2	<1.3
35–50	<20	<25	>18:30	>16:30	<1.1	<1.2
55–70	<15	<20	>21	>19	<0.9	<1.0

Note. These standards are for fitness programs. People wanting to do well in endurance performance need higher levels. Those at the *Good* level should emphasize maintaining this level the rest of their lives. Those in the lower levels should emphasize setting and reaching realistic goals.
[a]CRF declines with age.
[b]Women have lower standards because they have a larger amount of essential fat.

Reprinted, by permission, from E.T. Howley and B.D. Franks, 1986, *Health Fitness Instructor's Handbook.* (Champaign, IL: Human Kinetics), 85.

recommend that you try to achieve and maintain the "good" value for your age group; if you are not at that level, however, plan on making small and systematic progress toward that goal using the walking and jogging programs outlined in chapter 10.

Graded Exercise Tests

The field tests already mentioned are "all-out" tests in that you are asked to walk or run as fast as you can. Many fitness centers now offer a submaximal test of CRF that does not require an all-out effort. In such a test you might walk on a treadmill, step up and down on a bench, or ride a stationary bicycle (cycle ergometer) through a series of progressively more difficult stages until you reach a predetermined end point. Most of these tests are stopped when your heart rate reaches 70 to 85 percent of your age-adjusted estimate of maximal heart rate, which is calculated by subtracting your age from 220.

Typically, heart rate and blood pressure measures and an estimate of your subjective effort are obtained at each stage of the test. The most common index of effort is the Rating of Perceived Exertion (RPE) shown in table 5.3. In this scale, higher scores reflect more intense perceptions of effort; for example, the expression "extremely hard" indicates near-maximal work.

Heart Rate

Figure 5.1 shows how some of this information is used. The heart rate data were collected during a submaximal treadmill test of a 37-year-old man whose estimated maximal heart rate was 183 beats per minute $(220 - 37 = 183)$. The test used a walking speed of three miles per hour, and the grade (elevation) of the treadmill was increased 2.5 percent after each two minutes of the test. The man's heart rate was plotted against the grade, and a solid line was drawn through the points up to the last heart rate value measured in the test (85 percent of maximal heart rate). At this stage the test was still submaximal. A dashed line was then drawn along the same path up to the man's estimated maximal heart rate (183 beats per minute). At this point another line was "dropped" to the lower axis of the graph to indicate what the man's maximal work level would have been had he reached this stage of the test. The lower axis of the graph indicates the percent grade of the treadmill and the MET value equal to that grade. In this way a *submaximal* test can be used to estimate *maximal* aerobic fitness.

Table 5.3

Rating of Perceived Exertion Scales

Original rating scale		CR10 scale		
6	No exertion at all	0	Nothing at all	"No P"
7	Extremely light	0.3		
8		0.5	Extremely weak	Just noticeable
9	Very light	1	Very weak	
10		1.5		
11	Light	2	Weak	Light
12		2.5		
13	Somewhat hard	3	Moderate	
14		4		
15	Hard (heavy)	5	Strong	Heavy
16		6		
17	Very hard	7	Very strong	
18		8		
		9		
19	Extremely hard	**10**	**Extremely strong "Max P"**	
20	Maximal exertion	11		
		⭥		
		●	Absolute maximum	Highest possible

Borg RPE Scale © Gunnar Borg, 1970, 1985, 1994, 1998.
Borg CR10 Scale © Gunnar Borg, 1981, 1982, 1998.

How does this submaximal test show changes in CRF that have resulted from a training program? Typically, the heart rate response is lower at any given stage of the test following an endurance training program. If your heart rate response is 150 beats per minute at 15 percent grade before training, the value for the same work level may be only 130 beats per minute after training. You may therefore need to complete another stage or two of the test before you reach your 85-percent-of-maximal heart-rate cutoff.

Blood Pressure

Your blood pressure is monitored during a graded exercise test to provide additional information about how you adjust to increasing work rates. Blood pressure is given as two separate scores. The

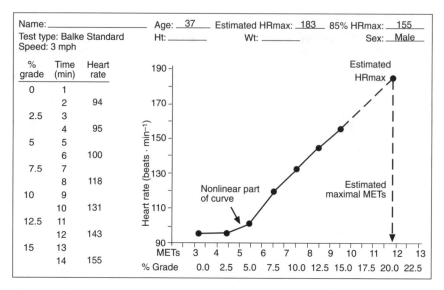

Figure 5.1 Maximal aerobic power estimated by measuring the heart rate response to a submaximal graded exercise test (GXT) on a treadmill

Reprinted, by permission, from E.T. Howley and B.D. Franks, 1997, *Health Fitness Instructor's Handbook*, 3d ed. (Champaign, IL: Human Kinetics), 222.

first and higher number is called *systolic blood pressure* and represents the highest pressure during a heartbeat; the second and lower number is *diastolic blood pressure* and is the pressure in the cardiovascular system when the heart is at rest. During a graded exercise test systolic pressure usually increases with each stage, while diastolic pressure decreases slightly or remains the same. If you do not respond in this manner, or if your systolic value becomes extremely high, the test is stopped before you achieve 85 percent of maximal.

Rating of Perceived Exertion

The RPE usually increases with each stage of a graded exercise test and is used as an indication of how close you may be to your maximum workload. Because your estimated maximal heart rate value is only an estimate and may actually be too high or too low, this is a good measure to obtain. Like any estimate, the formula 220 − age cannot predict each individual's maximal heart rate with exact precision (you have to do a maximal test to find your actual maximal heart rate). Because the estimate of maximal heart rate may be as much as 20 beats per minute too high or too low, the RPE score gives another indication of when you are reaching your personal end point.

How Many Calories Am I Using?

We have discussed how important modifications in both diet and exercise are in achieving weight-loss goals and maintaining the new weight (see chapter 3). Authorities often recommend that you burn 200 to 300 calories during each exercise session. Although most of us are familiar with the caloric costs of food, as values are usually printed on food packages, such is not the case for the caloric costs of physical activity. Since this is quite an important bit of information, researchers have developed various methods to measure the energy costs of physical activity.

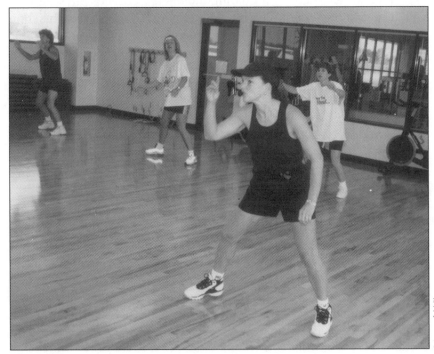

© Longenfeld Photo

Ways to Measure Energy Use

Oxygen is used to produce the energy needed to contract a muscle, initiate a nerve impulse, repair a bone, or carry out any number of cellular functions. Oxygen goes from the lungs to the blood and finally to the tissues where it is used. For each liter of oxygen used, the body produces about five calories of energy. Knowing this, it is possible to measure the amount of energy produced during the course of a day simply by measuring oxygen consumption. On the basis of these measurements we are able to estimate the amount of energy a person uses for different activities and provide an overall estimate of what a person might expend in one day.

When we are sitting at rest we expend about one calorie per hour for every kilogram (2.2 pounds) of body weight. The value of one calorie per kilogram per hour is one resting metabolic unit or 1 MET. METs have already been used to quantify your CRF. METs are also used in expressing the energy costs of activities; for example, running at six miles per hour requires 10 METs, or 10 times the rate of energy expended at rest. Before discussing the energy costs of physical activity, however, we need to focus on the energy associated with sitting at rest, the largest energy-producing task in the lives of most people! Given that we produce about one calorie of energy per kilogram of body weight per hour at rest, you can estimate your resting energy expenditure (also called basal metabolic rate, or BMR) by doing the following:

1. Multiply 24 calories by your body weight in kilograms (pounds divided by 2.2) or
2. Multiply 11 calories by your body weight in pounds

For example, for a 150-pound person, 150 pounds · 11 calories per pound = 1,650 calories. This, of course, represents only resting energy expenditure. To obtain an estimate of overall energy expenditure, you must add the energy cost of your other activities. This is done by adding from 400 to 800 calories, depending on whether you are sedentary or very active. So, if our 150-pound person is sedentary, the estimated total energy expenditure is 2,050 calories per day (1,650 calories + 400 calories).

Remember that this is a rough estimate and like any estimate, it may be too high or too low for you. Use it as a guide, but if you find yourself gaining weight even though you are eating just enough food

ESTIMATE YOUR DAILY ENERGY EXPENDITURE

1. Determine resting metabolic rate:

   Multiply 11 by your body weight:

   11 · _____ pounds = _____ calories

2. Select 400 calories if sedentary, 600 calories if moderately active, and 800 calories if active

3. Daily energy expenditure:

   Total from line 1: _____ calories + selection from

   line 2: _____ calories = _____ calories

to meet your estimated energy expenditure, decrease your estimate by about 10 percent and see if you can maintain weight on that new estimate. Keep in mind that if you reduce your caloric intake to a very low level, your body responds by decreasing its resting metabolic rate to protect its limited energy stores. In such a circumstance the above formula will result in an overestimation of energy expenditure.

Energy Costs of Common Activities

The techniques used to measure energy expenditure at rest have also been used to measure the energy required to do certain activities. This section presents information on the energy required for some of the most common activities associated with physical fitness programs.

Walking

We recommend a walking program for anyone who has not been active for some time. The program provides stages of gradually increasing duration and intensity and can be a lead-in to a jogging or running program. For many people a walking program may be all they want or need to maintain fitness. Walking has the advantage that it can be done anywhere, at any time, by virtually anyone.

Scientists have studied the energy cost of walking indoors using a treadmill and outdoors on a track, beach, or farm. Walking on a beach or across a plowed field requires more energy than walking at the same speed on a flat, firm surface. Because most people exercise on a firm surface, however, we will discuss the energy costs of walking with reference to this situation.

Table 5.4 shows the energy required to walk at different speeds with values given in calories per minute. Not surprisingly, the energy cost of walking increases with the speed of walking; however, the rate of increase is higher at the higher speeds. For example, when walking speed increases from two to three miles per hour for a 150-pound person, the energy required increases from 2.8 to 3.7 calories per minute. But going from four to five miles per hour requires an increase from 5.6 to 9 calories per minute. The energy cost of walking (or jogging or running, as we'll see later) also increases with the weight of the individual. As you can see in table 5.4, the 110-pound person expends fewer calories per minute compared with the 140-pound person at any given speed.

As we mentioned earlier, walking can be done by just about anyone to have a fitness effect. The very sedentary individual can walk at

Table 5.4
Energy Costs of Walking (kcal/Minute)

Body weight (lb)	MILES PER HOUR						
	2.0	2.5	3.0	3.5	4.0	4.5	5.0
110	2.1	2.4	2.8	3.1	4.1	5.2	6.6
120	2.3	2.6	3.0	3.4	4.4	5.6	7.2
130	2.5	2.9	3.2	3.6	4.8	6.1	7.8
140	2.7	3.1	3.5	3.9	5.2	6.6	8.4
150	2.8	3.3	3.7	4.2	5.6	7.0	9.0
160	3.0	3.5	4.0	4.5	5.9	7.5	9.6
170	3.2	3.7	4.2	4.8	6.3	8.0	10.2
180	3.4	4.0	4.5	5.0	6.7	8.4	10.8
190	3.6	4.2	4.7	5.3	7.0	8.9	11.4
200	3.8	4.4	5.0	5.6	7.4	9.4	12.0
210	4.0	4.6	5.2	5.9	7.8	9.9	12.6
220	4.2	4.8	5.5	6.2	8.2	10.3	13.2

Note. Multiply value by the duration of activity to obtain total calories expended.

moderate speeds to elevate the heart rate to the training zone needed for cardiovascular improvement, while the relatively fit individual can walk at high speeds to drive the heart rate to the right level.

Jogging and Running

Many people jog and run to achieve their fitness and weight-loss goals. The energy requirement of jogging is more than that of walking at three miles per hour, but is nearly the same as walking at five miles per hour. Table 5.5 shows the energy required to jog or run at different speeds. As you can see, the energy requirement increases with increasing speed, but the increase in the energy cost from one speed to the next is similar at slow and fast speeds, about 1.7 calories per minute per mile per hour. This proportional increase in energy cost means that when you jog a mile at six miles per hour (10 minutes per mile), you will finish the mile twice as fast as when jogging at three miles per hour, but the energy required per mile is about the same. We will discuss this topic further in the next section.

Table 5.5

Energy Costs of Jogging and Running (kcal/Minute)

Body weight (lb)	MILES PER HOUR							
	3.0	4.0	5.0	6.0	7.0	8.0	9.0	10.0
110	4.7	5.9	7.2	8.5	9.8	11.1	12.3	13.6
120	5.1	6.4	7.9	9.3	10.6	12.1	13.4	14.8
130	5.5	7.0	8.6	10.0	11.5	13.1	14.6	16.1
140	5.9	7.5	9.2	10.8	12.4	14.1	15.7	17.3
150	6.4	8.1	9.9	11.6	13.3	15.1	16.8	18.5
160	6.8	8.6	10.5	12.4	14.2	16.1	17.9	19.8
170	7.2	9.1	11.2	13.1	15.1	17.1	19.1	21.0
180	7.6	9.7	11.8	13.9	15.9	18.1	20.2	22.2
190	8.1	10.2	12.5	14.7	16.8	19.1	21.3	23.5
200	8.5	10.8	13.2	15.4	17.7	20.1	22.4	24.7
210	8.9	11.3	13.8	16.2	18.6	21.1	23.5	25.9
220	9.3	11.8	14.5	17.0	19.5	22.2	24.7	27.2

Note. Multiply value by the duration of activity to obtain total calories expended.

Caloric Costs of Walking Versus Running One Mile

In spite of the vast amount of information available regarding the energy costs of walking and running, a good deal of misunderstanding exists. We still hear claims that the energy cost of walking one mile is equal to that of running the same distance. Although this is generally not the case, walking can be just about as good as running for expending calories. We will try to explain this apparent contradiction.

Table 5.6 shows the energy cost of walking one mile, and table 5.7 shows the energy cost of running one mile. Given that energy cost is dependent on body weight (heavier people require more energy to travel one mile than lighter people do), the caloric cost is given for different body weights. The tables contain two numbers for each weight, one expressing the gross cost of the activity and the other expressing the net cost. Gross cost includes the resting metabolic rate (the cost of just sitting around), while net cost subtracts out this quantity. For weight-control programs it is important to use the net cost of an activity since it measures the energy used over and above that of sitting around.

Table 5.6

Gross and Net (Gross/Net) Cost in kcal per Mile for Walking

Body weight (lb)	MILES PER HOUR						
	2.0	2.5	3.0	3.5	4.0	4.5	5.0
110	64/39	58/39	54/39	53/39	60/48	68/57	79/69
120	69/42	63/42	59/42	57/42	66/52	75/63	86/75
130	75/45	68/45	64/45	62/45	71/57	81/68	93/81
140	80/49	73/49	69/49	67/49	77/61	87/73	100/88
150	87/52	79/52	74/52	72/52	82/65	93/78	108/94
160	92/56	84/56	79/56	76/56	88/70	100/84	115/100
170	98/59	90/59	84/59	81/59	93/74	106/89	122/107
180	104/63	95/63	89/63	86/63	99/78	112/94	129/113
190	110/66	100/66	94/66	91/66	104/83	118/99	136/119
200	115/70	105/70	99/70	95/70	110/87	124/104	144/125
210	121/73	111/73	104/73	100/73	115/92	131/110	151/132
220	127/77	116/77	109/77	105/77	121/96	137/115	158/138

Note. Multiply value by the number of miles walked to obtain the total (gross/net) calories expended.

Table 5.7

Gross and Net (Gross/Net) Cost
in kcal per Mile for Jogging and Running

Body weight (lb)	MILES PER HOUR							
	3.0	**4.0**	**5.0**	**6.0**	**7.0**	**8.0**	**9.0**	**10.0**
110	93/77	89/77	86/77	84/77	84/77	83/77	82/77	81/77
120	101/83	97/83	94/83	92/83	92/83	90/83	89/83	89/83
130	110/90	105/90	102/90	100/90	99/90	98/90	97/90	96/90
140	118/97	113/97	110/97	108/97	107/97	106/97	104/97	104/97
150	127/104	121/104	118/104	115/104	114/104	113/104	112/104	111/104
160	135/111	129/111	125/111	123/111	122/111	121/111	119/111	119/111
170	144/118	137/118	133/118	131/118	130/118	128/118	127/118	126/118
180	152/125	146/125	141/125	138/125	137/125	136/125	134/125	133/125
190	161/132	154/132	149/132	146/132	145/132	143/132	141/132	141/132
200	169/139	162/139	157/139	154/139	153/139	151/139	149/139	148/139
210	177/146	170/146	165/146	161/146	160/146	158/146	156/146	155/146
220	186/153	178/153	173/153	169/153	168/153	166/153	164/153	163/153

Note. Multiply value by the number of miles jogged or run to obtain the total (gross/net) calories expended.

When moving at slow to moderate speeds (2 to 3.5 miles per hour), the net cost of walking a mile is about half that of jogging or running a mile. This means that the person who jogs a mile at three miles per hour will be working at twice the metabolic rate of someone who walks at the same speed, and, of course, the heart rate response will be higher as well. Most people who walk move at these slower speeds, and so their energy cost per mile is half that of running.

Very high walking speeds of five miles per hour (one mile in 12 minutes), however, will result in a net energy cost similar to that of jogging or running. The heart-rate response of people walking at this speed may actually be higher than it would be if they were running at the same speed. If you can walk at these high speeds, you can easily reach your training heart rate and expend calories at about the same rate as during running.

You may now wonder why we stated that walking can be just about as good as jogging in expending calories. When a person jogs or runs, it takes time to leave the office or home, change clothes, gradually warm up, shower afterward, change clothes again, and return to the office or home. Of the 60 minutes that may be dedicated to a workout, only about 30 minutes may actually be spent running; the remainder is spent somewhat near the resting level. A person who walks for exercise can simply get up, perhaps change shirts, and get moving. Almost the entire 60 minutes is spent in activity. What this means is that although the net energy cost of walking is about half that of running, if the person who walks spends twice as much time walking as the other person spends running, the net energy expenditure for the two workouts is about the same!

Table 5.7 shows that the net caloric cost of running a mile is independent of speed. It does not matter whether you jog the mile at three miles per hour or run it at six miles per hour—caloric cost is the same. Obviously, it is going to take twice as long to run one mile at three miles per hour as at six miles per hour, but again, the net cost is about the same. There is no question that at six miles per hour you expend energy at about twice the rate seen at three miles per hour, but since the mile is finished in half the time, total energy expenditure is about the same. The heart-rate response will, of course, be higher during the six-mile-per-hour run.

Another point about the costs of walking and running a mile regards the actual number of calories expended per mile. A person weighing 154 pounds (70 kilograms) expends about 54 and 107 calories as a result of walking and running a mile, respectively. If this formerly sedentary person walks four miles a day, the additional energy expended above resting is 216 calories (4 · 54), and when coupled with a reduction in caloric intake of 300 calories a day, the person will experience about a one-pound loss of fat per week (500 kcal · 7 days = 3,500 kcal).

Before you take that next handful of potato chips, think in terms of how many miles it will take to "burn them off." One should not justify a milkshake by walking just one mile. Remember, it is the small, systematic changes you make in your diet and exercise habits that lead to weight loss and allow you to maintain the weight once you have achieved your goal.

One final comment about the energy costs of walking and running: as you lose weight, the energy your body requires to walk or run one mile decreases—there is simply less of you to carry around. This may help explain why some people experience a leveling off of body weight even though they are careful to keep the distance of their walks or runs the same during a weight-loss program. Knowing this, you should increase the distance you cover as you lose weight to keep up the same rate of weight loss.

Walking and running are not the only activities you can use in exercise programs to achieve fitness goals and to expend calories. We will now discuss bicycling, exercising to music, rope skipping, and swimming. In addition, a summary table will be presented at the end of the chapter to tie things together.

Bicycling

Bicycling is a more efficient form of human movement than walking or running. Consequently, you have to pedal more miles than you would have to walk to expend the same amount of energy. In general, you have to bicycle about two to three miles to expend the same number of calories as you would walking one mile. As most people can comfortably ride a bike at six to nine miles per hour, they can accomplish the same energy expenditure goal and take no more time than the person who walks at three miles per hour.

Exercising to Music

One popular form of exercise in fitness facilities and at home is exercising to music ("aerobics"). The intensity of the session depends on the type of activities being done—flexibility, muscular endurance, or cardiovascular. In addition, energy expenditure is dependent on whether a person walks through the exercises or does low-, moderate-, or high-intensity routines. The energy requirement for exercising to music, as shown in table 5.8, is as low as 3.3 METs for someone who participates in a low-intensity session (about the same as walking at 3.5 miles per hour), to as high as 10 METs in an a high-intensity session (about the same as jogging or running at six miles per hour).

As in walking and running, you need to be realistic about just how many calories are expended during this form of activity. If a 132-pound (60-kilogram) woman works at an average of 5 METs for an entire 40-minute session, she will expend 200 calories, equal to walking four miles. Given that she is making gains in cardiovascular fitness, flexibility, and muscular endurance, this is a very reasonable number of calories to expend. Because these exercises involve small muscle groups and require other muscles to stabilize body positions, heart-rate responses tend to be elevated at any level of energy expenditure compared to walking or jogging.

Table 5.8

Gross Energy Cost of Exercising to Music (kcal per Minute)

Body weight (lb)	Low intensity	Moderate intensity	High intensity
110	3.3	5.8	8.3
120	3.6	6.4	9.1
130	3.9	6.9	9.8
140	4.2	7.4	10.6
150	4.5	7.9	11.3
160	4.8	8.5	12.1
170	5.1	9.0	12.8
180	5.4	9.5	13.6
190	5.7	10.1	14.3
200	6.0	10.6	15.1
210	6.3	11.1	15.9
220	6.6	11.7	16.7

Note. Multiply value by the duration of activity to obtain total calories expended.

Rope Skipping

Rope skipping can be done indoors or out, requires little formal equipment, and can be an effective component of a fitness program for people with high levels of fitness and regular activity. We emphasize the latter point because rope skipping places a load primarily on the lower leg, involves smaller muscle groups than walking and running do, and causes a disproportionately higher heart-rate response.

Overdoing this activity, especially if you are at the beginning of a fitness program, is inappropriate. Our concern is based on the energy cost of rope skipping (see table 5.9). Even a very slow skipping rate (60 to 80 turns per minute) requires 9 METs and a heart rate of more than 150 beats per minute in young, fit subjects. Skipping at 120 turns per minute increases the energy cost to only 11 METs. As a result, skipping is not a "graded" activity—even the slowest skipping rate (60 to 80 turns per minute) for an extended period requires an energy expenditure equal to or higher than the cardiorespiratory fitness of many sedentary people.

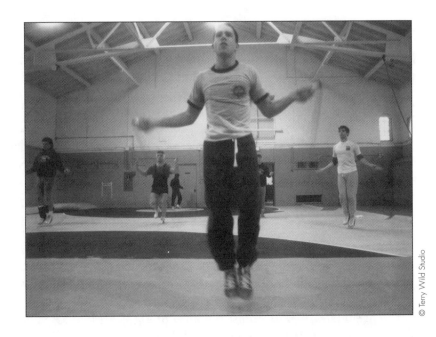

Table 5.9

Gross Energy Cost of Rope Skipping
(kcal per Minute)

Body weight (lb)	Slow skipping	Fast skipping
110	7.5	9.2
120	8.2	10.0
130	8.9	10.9
140	9.5	11.7
150	10.2	12.5
160	10.9	13.4
170	11.6	14.2
180	12.3	15.0
190	13.0	15.9
200	13.6	16.7
210	14.3	17.5
220	15.0	18.4

Note. Multiply value by the duration of activity to obtain total calories expended.

Swimming

Swimming is an excellent activity because it involves the large muscle groups and provides little trauma to joints while expending a relatively large number of calories. However, predicting the caloric cost of swimming is difficult because it depends on the type of stroke used, the swimming speed, and the skill of the swimmer. A poor swimmer must expend greater quantities of energy just to stay afloat or move at a slow pace, while a highly skilled swimmer expends very few calories doing the same thing. As a rule, the net caloric cost of swimming one mile has been estimated to be about four times that of running one mile (400 kcal vs. 100 kcal).

Table 5.10 shows the estimated caloric cost per mile of swimming the front crawl for men and women. Because of their greater buoyancy associated with higher body fatness, women expend fewer calories per mile than men, independent of skill level. It should be noted that the maximal heart rate is about 13 beats per minute lower in water than on land. For this reason your training heart rate for swimming is about 10 beats per minute lower than your value for running or cycling.

Energy Costs of Physical Activities

We have presented only a few of the most common activities used in fitness programs. Table 5.11 provides details about other activities you may choose for your own fitness program. The MET level gives

Table 5.10

Caloric Cost Per Mile (kcal per Mile) of Swimming the Front Crawl for Men and Women by Skill Level

Skill level	Women	Men
Competitive	180	280
Skilled	260	360
Average	300	440
Unskilled	360	560
Poor	440	720

Note. Multiply value by number of miles to obtain total calories expended.

Adapted from Holmer, 1979.

Table 5.11

Summary of Measured Energy Cost
of Various Physical Activities

Activity	METs kcal/kg/hr	KCAL/HR 50 kg/ 110 lbs	70 kg/ 154 lbs	90 kg/ 198 lbs
Archery	3.5	175	245	315
Backpacking (general)	7	350	490	630
Badminton (social)	4.5	225	315	405
Badminton (competitive)	7	350	490	630
Basketball (game)	8	400	560	720
Basketball (general)	6	300	420	540
Billiards	2.5	125	175	225
Bowling	3	150	210	270
Boxing (in ring)	12	600	840	1080
Canoeing (moderate)	7	350	490	630
Canoeing (vigorous)	12	600	840	1080
Cricket	5	250	350	450
Croquet	2.5	125	175	225
Cycling (light)	6	300	420	540
Cycling (moderate)	8	400	560	720
Cycling (vigorous)	10	500	700	900
Dancing (ballroom, slow)	3	150	210	270
Dancing (ballroom, fast)	5.5	275	385	495
Dancing (aerobic)		see table 5.8		
Fencing	6	300	420	540
Field hockey	8	400	560	720
Fishing (general)	4	200	280	360
Fishing (in waders)	6	300	420	540
Football (touch)	8	400	560	720
Golf (pulling clubs)	5	250	350	450
Golf (carrying clubs)	5.5	275	385	495
Golf (power cart)	3.5	175	245	315
Handball (general)	12	600	840	1080
Hiking	6	300	420	540
Horseback riding (trotting)	6.5	325	455	585
Horseshoe pitching	3	150	210	270
Hunting (general)	5	250	350	450
Jogging		see tables 5.5, 5.7		
Paddle/racquetball, general	6.5	325	455	585
Paddle/raquetball, competitive	10	500	700	900
Rock climbing, ascending	11	550	770	990

(continued)

Table 5.11 *(continued)*

Activity	METs kcal/kg/hr	KCAL/HR 50 kg/ 110 lbs	70 kg/ 154 lbs	90 kg/ 198 lbs
Rope jumping		see table 5.9		
Running		see tables 5.5, 5.7		
Sailing (general)	3	150	210	270
Scuba diving (general)	7	350	490	630
Shuffleboard	3	150	210	270
Skating, roller and ice	7	350	490	630
Sledding	7	350	490	630
Snowshoeing	8	400	560	720
Squash	12	600	840	1080
Soccer (general)	7	350	490	630
Soccer (competitive)	10	500	700	900
Swimming		see table 5.10		
Table tennis (general)	7	350	490	630
Tennis (general)	7	350	490	630
Volleyball (general)	3	150	210	270
Walking		see tables 5.4, 5.6		

Note. Values from: Ainsworth, B.E., Haskell, W.L., Leon, A.S., Jacobs, D.S., Jr., Montoye, H.J., Sallis, J.F., and Paffenbarger, R.S., Jr. (1993). Compendium of physical activities: Classification by energy costs of human physical activities. *Medicine and Science in Sports and Exercise*, 25, 71–80.

some indication of the relative intensity of each activity and should provide some guidance as to whether you should include it in your activity program. Remember to select activities consistent with your fitness level and do the activity long enough to achieve your caloric-expenditure goal. Caloric expenditures are listed for three body weights, indicating an approximate range of energy expenditures associated with each activity.

At this point, you know how to use walk/run tests to evaluate CRF. If you have your CRF evaluated with a graded exercise test, you know how the fitness instructor determines your value. Finally, the information on how many calories you use during exercise should help you achieve weight-loss and weight-maintenance goals.

chapter **6**

Flexibility and Stretching

Flexibility is a measure of how well a joint moves through its normal range of motion. For example, starting with your arms held straight at your sides, can you raise your arms out to the side and up until your hands touch high over your head? If you can, you have a normal range of motion (flexibility) in your shoulder joints.

Each joint has a limited range of motion related to its structure and the tissues surrounding it. It is important to maintain the flexibility of each joint so that normal everyday tasks can be completed without undue strain. Lack of flexibility can be related to medical problems, with low back pain being one example.

Lack of Flexibility

Flexibility, like any trait, is limited by our genetic endowment. It is clear, however, that regular use is necessary to develop and maintain that endowment. For example, when a cast is removed from someone who had a broken bone at the elbow joint, that person's initial attempts to move the joint through its normal range of motion are usually painful and not very successful. What causes the lack of flexibility at the elbow joint? While the arm is immobilized in the cast, fibrous connective tissue, or "adhesions," begin to cling to the tendons, ligaments, and bones in the joint, reducing its range of motion. In addition, due to the fact that the cast holds the arm at a fixed angle, the upper arm muscles become shortened and do not allow the arm to straighten when the cast is removed. Flexibility, then, is affected by both the condition of the connective tissues at the joint and the ability of the muscle to stretch. Stretching exercises are aimed at lengthening muscles and reducing the development of inappropriate connective tissues at the joint, thereby maintaining a normal range of motion.

Improving Flexibility

If you want to improve your flexibility, you must stretch beyond your current range of motion. In addition, if you don't perform stretching exercises, you will lose some of the flexibility you presently have. Finally, improvements in flexibility are specific to the muscles and joints involved in the stretching exercises. Consequently, a stretching program improves overall flexibility one joint at a time.

The two major types of stretching exercises are *static* and *dynamic* (ballistic). In static stretching you *slowly* stretch a muscle group, hold

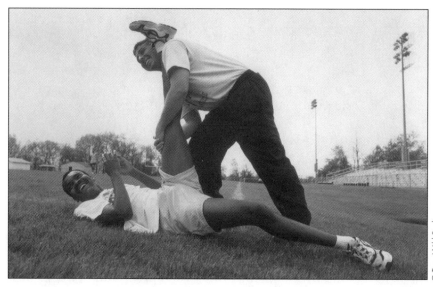

© Terry Wild Studio

the stretch at the point of mild tension, and then relax. You may hold the stretch for only 10 seconds at the beginning of your stretching program and increase to 30 seconds with practice. The static stretching technique has been shown to be successful in accomplishing flexibility goals with little chance of causing problems. Ballistic stretching is the "bouncy" stretching that you see when someone is having difficulty touching his or her toes. Ballistic stretching can be counterproductive. When a muscle is suddenly lengthened, as happens in "bouncing," the muscle responds with a reflex contraction. This is the opposite of the intended effect of stretching exercises.

In static stretching:

1. Hold stretches to the point of mild tension, not pain.
2. Breathe normally during each stretching exercise. Do not hold your breath.
3. Do each exercise slowly.

Including Stretching in Your Workout

You should include specific stretching exercises as a regular part of your warm-up and cool-down in each workout. These stretching exercises, along with other warm-up activities, help prepare your joints for the more strenuous dynamic activity to come by releasing fluids that lubricate the joint and by increasing the size of the joint's soft cartilage, which absorbs the shock of impact associated with normal physical activity. Used during cool-down, stretching exercises help maintain and improve flexibility. In addition, stretching exercises help ease the transition from the resting state to the exercise state and from exercise back to rest.

Using a variety of stretching exercises will help maintain the function of as many joints as possible. The recommended stretching exercises start at the neck and proceed downward. Each is done *slowly* and is held for 10 to 30 seconds. Each of the exercises can be repeated two or three times. In addition to static stretches, you can do controlled dynamic movements to get the body ready for more strenuous activity.

Fitness participants often ask whether they should do static stretching before or after warming up. The reason behind warming up first is that the muscles and other tissues are easier to stretch when they are warm. The other side of the argument is that muscles are normally "warm," and light warm-up activities don't affect that very much. We recommend that you do some light stretching activities before you begin and a more thorough program of stretching during your cool-down when your body temperature is elevated.

Stretching Exercises

The following figures and instructions provide a comprehensive series of stretches you can use to improve your flexibility and aid in your warm-up and cool-down.

NECK

Neck Stretch

While sitting or standing with your head in its normal upright position, slowly tilt it to the right until tension is felt on the left side of your neck. Hold that tension for 10 to 30 seconds and then return your head to the upright position. Repeat to the left side, and then toward the front. Always return to the upright position before moving on.

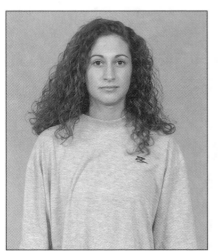 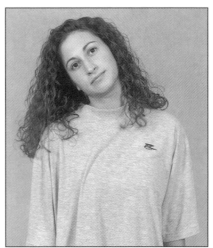

SHOULDERS

Reach to the Sky

Stand with feet shoulder-width apart. Raise both arms overhead so that your hands are intertwined, palms facing. Hold for 10 to 30 seconds and relax.

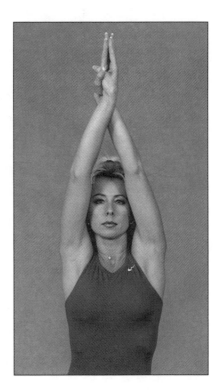

Reach Back

Stand with feet shoulder-width apart and hold your arms out to the sides with thumbs pointing down. Slowly move both arms back until you feel tension. Hold for 10 to 30 seconds and relax.

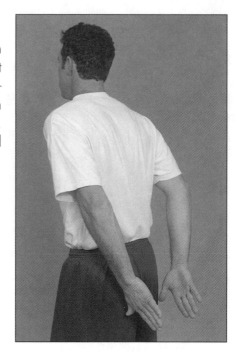

Arm Circles

Stand with feet shoulder-width apart and hold arms straight out to the side with your palms facing up. Start moving your arms slowly in small circles and gradually make larger and larger circles. Come back to the starting position and reverse the direction of your arm swing.

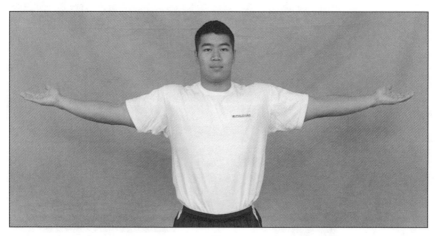

TRUNK

Side Bend

Stand with feet shoulder-width apart and place your hands on your waist. Slowly bend to the right side until you feel tension. Hold for 10 to 30 seconds and relax. Repeat on the other side.

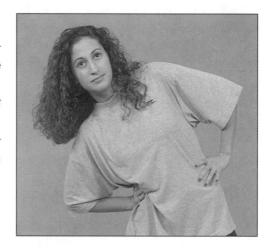

Sit and Twist

Sit on a mat with your left leg straight in front of you. Bend your right leg and cross it over your left leg so that your right foot is alongside your left knee. Bring your left elbow across your body and place it on the outside of your right thigh near the knee. Slowly twist your body as you look over your right shoulder. Your left elbow should be exerting pressure against your right thigh. Hold the stretch for 10 to 30 seconds, relax, and repeat for the other side.

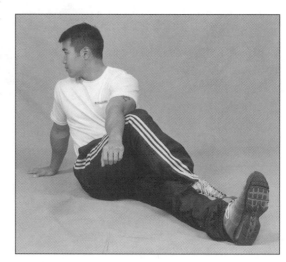

Knee to Chest

Lie on your back on a mat with your legs straight. Bend your left knee and bring it up toward your chest. Grasp the underside of your thigh and slowly pull your thigh to your chest. Hold for 10 to 30 seconds. Release, and repeat with the right leg.

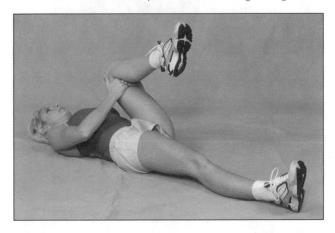

GROIN

Groin Stretch

Sit on a mat with your knees bent. Put the soles of your feet (or shoes) together and hold onto your ankles. Place your elbows on the inner sides of your knees and slowly apply downward pressure until you feel tension. Hold for 10 to 30 seconds and repeat.

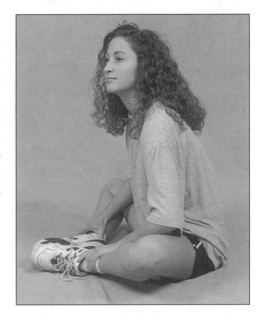

LEGS

Lying Quad Stretch

Lie on your stomach and grasp your right ankle with your right hand. Slowly bring it up until you feel tension on the front side of your thigh. Hold for 10 to 30 seconds and repeat with the left leg.

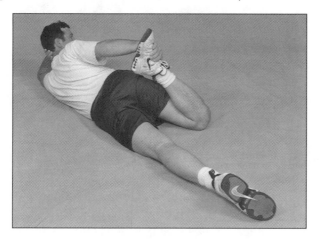

Hamstring Stretch

While standing, raise your right foot onto a table, bench, or chair so that your leg is almost parallel to the floor. Slowly move your hands along your right leg toward your ankle until you feel tension on the underside of the thigh. Hold the tension for 10 to 30 seconds and relax. Repeat for the other leg. See the modified hurdler's stretch on page 109 for another hamstring stretch.

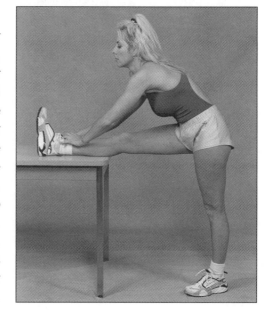

Achilles Stretch

Stand facing a wall with your left foot close to the wall and your left knee bent. With your right leg straight, slowly lean toward the wall, *keeping your right heel flat on the ground.* Hold for 10 to 30 seconds and relax. Repeat for the left leg.

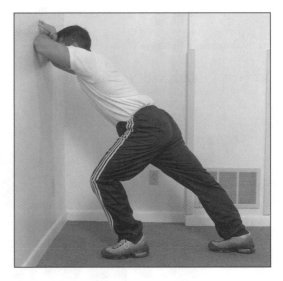

Healthy Low Back

Low back pain is one of the most common complaints among adults in the United States. Low back problems account for more lost person hours than any other type of occupational injury and are the most frequent cause of activity limitation in U.S. citizens under age 45. If you have never had low back problems, be grateful and include some daily preventive exercises to help reduce the chance that the problem will occur.

Causes of Low Back Pain

Many factors are related to low back problems, including structural abnormalities, some diseases, accidents, inappropriate lifting, poor posture, lack of warm-up prior to vigorous activity, lack of abdominal strength and endurance, lack of flexibility in the back and legs, and an inability to cope with stress. You should call your doctor if

- the pain continues for about a month,
- you are less than 25 or above 55 years old,
- you have or have had cancer,
- the pain has resulted from serious injury or trauma,
- the pain becomes worse when you lie down,

- you can't walk,
- you have fever with pain,
- you have numbness of the extremities, or
- you are experiencing defecation and urination problems.

FACTS ON LOW BACK PAIN

- Ninety percent of adults in the United States will have a back problem during their lifetime.
- Low back pain is responsible for one-third of all disability dollars, about $24 billion in the United States.
- In 84 percent of cases no definite cause is found. Disc herniation, found only in 5 percent of the remaining cases, usually resolves spontaneously without surgical intervention.
- Continuous sitting, lying down, and the use of strong painkillers such as narcotics are the worst things one can do for back pain.
- The best thing one can do for preventing and treating low back pain is to participate in an appropriate exercise program.

Structural Abnormalities

A very small percentage of low back problems are caused by anatomical problems (e.g., a deformed spine, one leg longer than the other). These conditions may be altered by a structural device or may require surgery.

Diseases

Some diseases, such as arthritis or tuberculosis of the spine, are directly related to the back and may result in back problems. Other diseases seemingly unrelated to the back can also result in back pain, including kidney or gall bladder disease, a urinary tract infection, cancer in the region, a peptic ulcer, a tipped uterus, or an ovarian infection.

Accidents

Many physical ailments, including low back problems, result from accidents. These problems often require long hours of rehabilitation to help the affected person return to a normal lifestyle.

Prevention of Back Problems

Although some of the factors discussed are generally not under your control, you can modify some factors associated with back pain. The way you move your body during everyday activities has a good deal to do with whether or not you develop back problems.

Lifting

People often injure their backs trying to lift objects that are too heavy or using poor lifting techniques. Figure 6.12 illustrates proper lifting techniques. Guidelines for proper lifting follow:

- Look at the object before you lift. Since its appearance and size may deceive you as to its weight, try to estimate the weight by gently pushing it with your hands or feet. Avoid lifting objects too heavy for you.
- Face the object and see if you can get a good grip.
- Use your leg muscles by bending your knees and keeping your back straight.
- Keep the object close to the center of your body in the space between your shoulder and waist.
- Do not arch your back when lifting an object. Use a ladder to reach objects over your head.
- Walk slowly and avoid uneven and slippery surfaces.
- If you are wearing a back belt to stabilize your back, do not rely on it and try to lift objects too heavy for you.

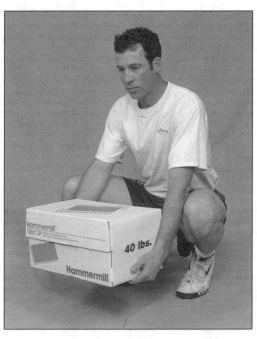

Figure 6.12 Proper lifting technique

Note. A load of 50 pounds held close to the body and lifted 4 inches from the floor will generate a compression force on the back in excess of 770 pounds. If the same load is held horizontally 12 inches from the body, it will increase this force to 924 pounds. Increasing the horizontal distance to 20 inches will increase the force to 1,106 pounds. According to the National Institute of Occupational Safety and Health (NIOSH), lifting to a vertical distance of approximately 36 inches from the floor is safe for all loads when the horizontal distance from the body is 20 inches or less.

Posture

Poor posture while sleeping, sitting, or standing can contribute to low back problems. The suggestions that follow may be helpful.

- While sitting and lying, avoid extremes in your posture; contrary to popular belief, a slight rounding of the back and shoulders is healthy.
- A small pillow placed at the lowest part of your back (just above the hips) when you are sitting or lying can help maintain the normal low back curve.
- Avoid rigid positions (e.g., military attention) and extreme hyper-extension (head and shoulders pressed back, knees locked).
- Sleeping on your stomach or on your back with legs straight tends to exaggerate the normal curve in your low back and may be a cause of low back pain or discomfort in some individuals.
- Sleeping on the side or on the back with knees bent appears to be comfortable and appropriate for most individuals.
- Putting a pillow between your legs when sleeping on your side will decrease the pressure on your back. (Your mattress can also be a factor; for example, a posture that results in discomfort on a firm mattress may not cause a problem on a water bed.)
- Carrying your wallet in one of your hip pockets will put pressure on your sciatic nerve and cause pain if you are sitting or driving for prolonged periods of time.
- Whenever possible, avoid prolonged standing, as it may cause fatigue in the supporting muscles of the trunk.
- Bending your knees slightly while standing, and shifting your weight with one foot slightly elevated during extended standing are ways to help prevent back problems.

Warming Up

Warming up can help to prevent low back problems. Using stretching and strengthening exercises for the midtrunk area (abdominal muscles, back, upper legs) as a regular part of your warm-up can help you develop the strength, endurance, and flexibility needed to prevent low back problems. One frequent low back problem is a strain that results from sudden or forceful bending or twisting while playing a game (e.g., racquetball). Warming up the muscles you will use in the activity before a game can help prevent this type of muscle strain.

Abdominal Strength and Endurance

Chapter 7 deals with total body muscular strength and endurance. Abdominal strength and endurance have been recognized as important to a healthy low back. The abdominal muscles play a major role in preventing an excessive forward tilt of the pelvis; strong abdominal muscles support the trunk in postures that otherwise could cause back problems. In forward-leaning postures, strong abdominal muscle contractions can decrease the stress placed on the back.

Many exercises that have been used in the past to strengthen the abdominal area actually appear to make the problem worse. These include straight-leg sit-ups, sit-ups performed with someone holding your feet, timed sit-ups, and double leg raises.

ABDOMEN

Curl-Up

The best type of exercise for the abdominal region is a slow curl-up with knees bent and feet flat but not held. The curl-up is the first part of a sit-up, but instead of coming all the way up to a sitting position, you stop at what is called the "sticking point." This is the point in the sit-up at which it would require additional effort—more muscle involvement—to come all the way up. Your abdominal muscles do the work during the curl-up stage, but you have to use additional muscles to go from the sticking point all the way up to a sit-up. Since we are most interested in working the abdominal muscles, a curl-up is the recommended exercise, unless it causes increased back pain. Do curl-ups slowly and increase the number done gradually over time until you can do a total of 30 to 40 each day.

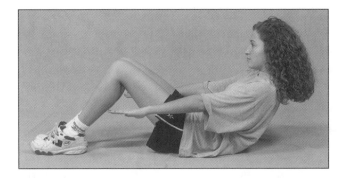

Diagonal Curl

To strengthen different parts of the abdominal muscles than those developed with the curl-up, alternate the diagonal curl to the left and to the right.

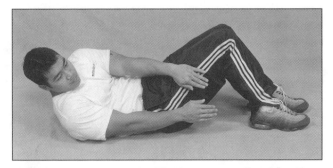

Pelvic Tilt

Lie on your back with knees bent, feet flat on the floor, and arms at your sides. Flatten the small of your back against the floor (which will cause your hips to tilt upward). Hold.

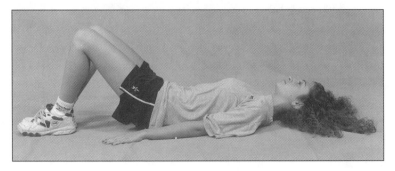

Flexibility

The first part of this chapter dealt with total body flexibility. An important component related to low back problems is the amount of flexibility you have in the low back and upper legs. The muscles that move the hips in different directions are associated with low back pain. Either lack of flexibility or lack of strength and endurance in this region can result in back problems. One way to deal with low back problems is to do static stretching, which involves slowly lengthening the muscle(s) to a point of slight discomfort; when you reach this point, hold the position for 10 to 30 seconds, with one or two repeats. Progressively increasing the range of motion results in improved flexibility.

LOW BACK

Hyperextension

Most low back stretches involve flexion of the back (moving forward). Some extension (moving backward) and slight hyperextension is recommended for most people. If you already have a back problem or you experience pain with hyperextension, seek medical advice. For most people, some hyperextension is recommended, but *don't* go as far as you can backward in the hyperextension.

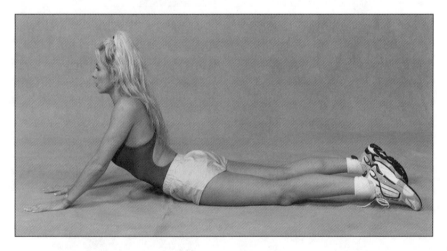

Modified Hurdler's Stretch

Whenever possible, do static stretching exercises sitting or lying down rather than standing. For example, it is better to sit with one leg out and the other flexed and stretch toward one's toes on the extended leg, as in the hurdler's stretch, than to do a standing toe touch.

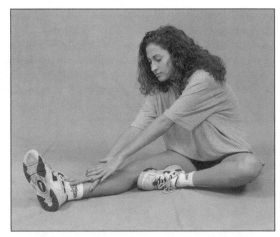

Back Extension

Slowly bend your body back at the waist as far as you can. If you experience any pain during this exercise, you should stop immediately. If the pain continues after you have stopped or if it reoccurs when you exercise again, inform your physician.

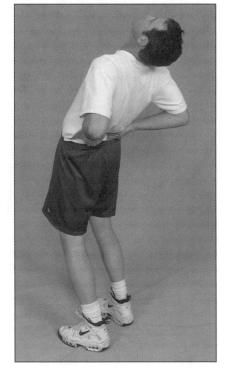

Knee-to-Chest Flexion

Bring your knees up toward your chest and hold, keeping your back flat on the floor.

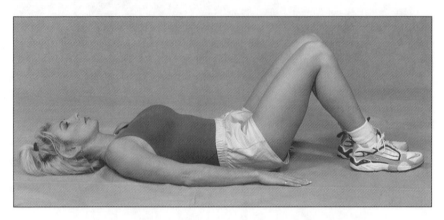

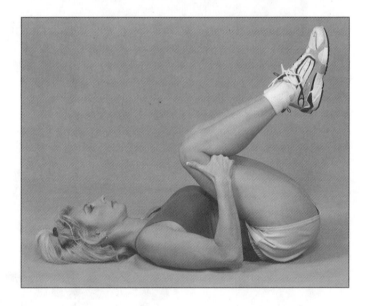

Trunk Flexion

Slowly bend forward and hold for 20–30 seconds.

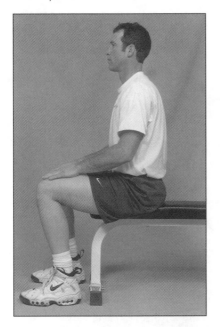

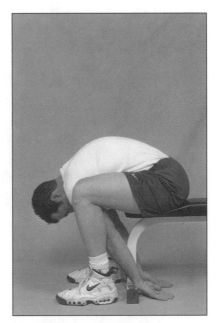

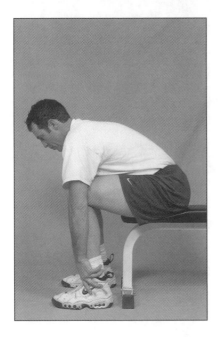

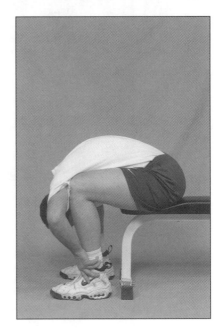

Back Flexibility

Kneel on all fours and raise first one arm and then the other arm. Next, raise one leg and then the other leg. Finally, raise the arm and leg from opposite sides and then repeat with the other arm and leg. Do all movements slowly and hold for a few seconds.

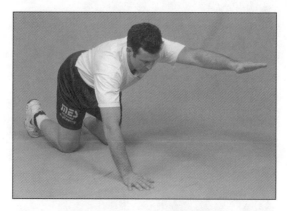

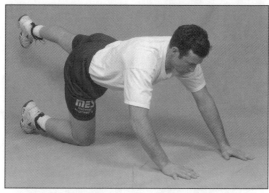

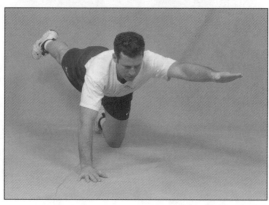

Trunk Arch

On your hands and knees, tuck in your chin and arch your back. Slowly sit back on your heels, letting your shoulders drop to the floor. Hold.

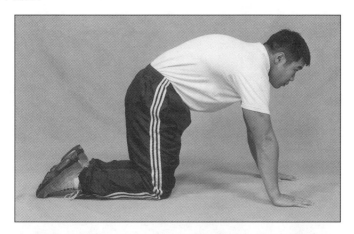

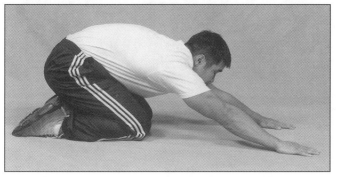

Cat and Camel

On your hands and knees with your head parallel to the floor, arch your back and then let it slowly sag toward the floor. Try to keep your arms straight.

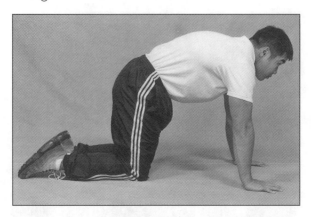

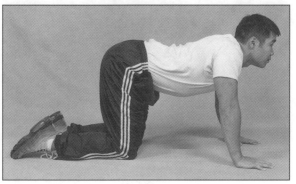

Coping With Stress

Although an inability to cope with stress will not cause back problems if your back is strong, it can cause problems in persons already at risk for back problems. Suggestions for coping with stress are included in chapter 9.

Flexibility is an important component of fitness. By adding stretching exercises to your fitness workout, you can increase your range of motion and lower your chances of injury, particularly to the low back. When we are flexible, we are able to comfortably enjoy exercise and easily accomplish a variety of daily tasks.

chapter 7

Muscular Strength and Endurance

M uscular strength describes the *maximum* force that can be generated by a muscle. A person with a great deal of strength can lift very heavy weights. Strength is dependent on the size of the muscle and the ability to "recruit" available muscle fibers, which is related to the individual's level of arousal. In contrast, muscular endurance describes the ability of a muscle to make repeated contractions against a *less-than-maximal* load. An individual who can lift a weight many times before experiencing fatigue has a high level of muscular endurance.

For many years, health-related fitness programs focused on participation in aerobic exercise to improve cardiorespiratory fitness and to expend calories to achieve a healthy body weight. Today's fitness programs broaden this focus to include exercises to improve muscular strength and endurance to achieve the following results.

• *Reduce the chance of osteoporosis.* Osteoporosis, a thinning of the bone that is related to fractures in the elderly, is a growing problem in our society as the "baby boomer" generation enters its sixth decade. Osteoporosis is the result of a reduction in estrogen that occurs at menopause, inadequate calcium intake (see chapter 4), and inadequate exercise and strength. The downward force associated with exercise in the standing position (e.g., weight-bearing activities such as walking or jogging) and the lateral forces exerted by muscle contractions help retain bone mass.

• *Maintain muscle mass.* Muscle mass also maintains the resting metabolic rate, the largest portion of our total daily energy expenditure. This helps prevent the weight gain that often occurs with age (see chapter 3).

• *Reduce the chance of low back pain.* Inadequate abdominal muscle strength and endurance make it more difficult to maintain the pelvis in its proper orientation, resulting in an exaggeration of the "curves" of the low back and subsequent back pain.

• *Reduce the effort required to perform activities of daily living.* Adequate muscular strength and endurance make the usual daily activities less strenuous and reduce the stress that might be transferred to weaker tissues when an individual can't lift a load properly.

• *Improve one's self-concept (confidence).* Lastly, individuals who are strong feel better about themselves. This alone justifies including muscular strength and endurance exercises as a regular part of your workouts.

Testing Muscular Strength

How strong are you? Your answer depends, in part, on the type of strength test you take. Strength is measured with isometric, isokinetic, and isotonic tests.

Isometric strength is measured with instruments such as the *grip dynamometer*, which measures the force of your grip, or the *cable tensiometer*, which measures the strength of most muscle groups. In an isometric contraction the muscle does not shorten (*isometric* means "constant length") even though the person is exerting maximal force. Isometric strength varies with the angle of the joint and does not provide a measure of strength throughout the normal range of motion of a joint.

Isokinetic strength is measured with a special machine that controls the speed at which you can move a joint through its range of motion. A limb, such as the lower leg, is attached to a lever arm that controls how fast the limb moves. When a muscle contracts with as much force as possible to move the limb, sensors in the machine monitor force throughout the range of motion. These machines are expensive and can usually be found in physical therapy and athletic training facilities.

Isotonic (dynamic) strength is the most familiar type of strength measure. Strength is simply measured as the heaviest weight lifted through a normal range of motion using either a barbell or a machine.

The greatest weight you can lift in good form through a joint's range of motion is called the one-repetition maximum, or 1-RM, and is a measure of maximal muscle strength. To measure your 1-RM, you are asked to lift a weight you think you can lift and then lift increasingly heavier weights only once each until you get to a weight you cannot lift. The last weight lifted in good form is your 1-RM. Some fitness facilities measure the 3-RM or 5-RM because it requires a less intense effort.

Testing Muscular Endurance

Muscular endurance is typically measured by counting the number of lifts you can do with a fixed weight. This is sometimes called *absolute muscular endurance*, as the weight that is lifted is a fixed (absolute) quantity. This approach can be used to show progress over time. A person might be able to do only five arm curls with a 25-pound weight prior to a training program but may increase that number to 20 after the program.

Another approach is to measure *relative muscular endurance*, which shows how many times you can lift a weight that is a certain percentage (e.g., 70 percent) of your 1-RM. Because the 1-RM (maximal strength) will change during a training program, this approach allows you to see how your muscular endurance changes as your strength increases. For example, at the beginning of a training program your 1-RM might be 60 pounds for an arm curl and you might lift 42 pounds (70 percent of 60 pounds) 10 times. At the end of the training program your 1-RM might be 80 pounds and you might lift 56 pounds (70 percent of 80 pounds) only six times. In this case muscular strength increased faster than muscular endurance.

Another way arm and shoulder strength and endurance can be measured is to use the modified pull-up. (See the figures at the top of page 127.) Since your feet support part of your weight, this test is more appropriate for many fitness participants than a standard pull-up, which requires you to lift your full weight. You can also use the

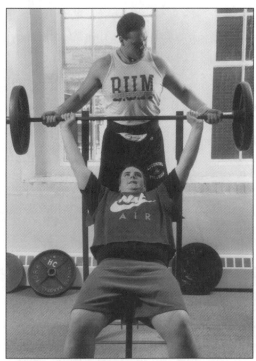

© Terry Wild Studio

90-degree push-up as a test of arm and shoulder strength and endurance. (See the figures at the top of page 126.)

Training Principles

The two guiding principles for planning exercise programs to improve muscular strength and endurance are *overload* and *specificity.* The overload principle states that to make improvements, a muscle must lift a weight heavier than that to which it is accustomed. As your muscles adapt to the new load, you must overload the muscles again to achieve additional strength gains.

The principle of specificity states that the type of adaptation (i.e., muscular strength or muscular endurance) is related to the type of exercise. If a person lifts heavy weights, the primary change is an increase in the size of the muscle cell, an adaptation called *hypertrophy.* This increase in muscle size is associated with the increase in muscle strength. On the other hand, if a person does many repetitions with lighter weights (e.g., 50 percent of 1-RM), the primary changes in muscle are found in the energy-producing parts, called mitochondria, and in the number of capillaries that bring oxygen to the muscle cell. Muscle size does not increase very much with endurance exercise. Though in general the effects of training are specific to the type of exercise performed, there is some overlap in the areas of strength and endurance because a person cannot completely isolate one from the other.

Strength increases over the course of a training program, but hypertrophy doesn't occur until later (more than 10 weeks) in the program. The strength gain early in the program comes primarily from neural changes related to coordination of the major muscle groups and the ability to recruit more muscle fibers. Men typically experience more hypertrophy than women as a result of a long-term training program. This is primarily because men have more testosterone, a hormone that has more anabolic (tissue-building) properties than estrogen.

Training Programs for Muscular Strength and Endurance

Progressive Resistance Exercise (PRE) is a general term that describes a method to progressively and systematically overload a muscle group.

A PRE program specifies both the weight (load) lifted and the maximum number of repetitions the load is lifted (RM). The term *set* describes the number of repetitions done before a rest period. For example, if you were to do three sets of a 10-RM routine, you would choose a weight you can lift a maximum of 10 times (10-RM) and do the following:

1. Lift weight 10 times; rest.
2. Lift weight 10 times; rest.
3. Lift weight 10 times; rest.

For gains in muscular *strength*, follow a 4- to 8-RM routine (choose a weight you can lift a maximum of four to eight times) and do three sets. When you can lift the weight more than eight times in each of two to three sets, increase the weight. In this way you are progressively increasing the load against which the muscles must work (the overload principle). For gains in muscular *endurance,* do three sets of a 15- to 30-RM routine. High repetitions with lighter weights result in specific muscular endurance adaptations. Weight training, like aerobics, should be done on an every-other-day basis.

Weight Training

The first question to ask in a weight training program is: how much weight should I start with? Two general guidelines follow:

1. For arm exercises, start your PRE program with a weight equal to one-fourth to one-third of your body weight. If you weigh 180 pounds, start with 45 (one-fourth of 180) to 60 (one-third of 180) pounds.
2. For leg exercises, start your PRE program with a weight equal to one-half to two-thirds of your body weight. If you weigh 180 pounds, start with 90 (one-half of 180) to 120 (two-thirds of 180) pounds.

Table 7.1 provides a summary of starting weights for people of different body weights.

Table 7.1

Starting Weights (in Pounds) for Weight Training for Arms and Legs

Body weight (lb)	Arms	Legs
100	25–33	50–67
120	30–40	60–80
140	35–46	70–93
160	40–53	80–107
180	45–60	90–120
200	50–66	100–133

Remember, in choosing a starting point in your PRE program, *it is better to do too little than too much.* You can use the selected weight training activities in the following section to increase muscular strength and endurance. Similar exercises can be done using machine weights.

To maximize safety, follow these guidelines:

- Warm up before exercise and cool down after exercise.

- Work with a "spotter" for free-weight workouts to prevent being trapped under a weight (such as the bench press).

- Use collars for plate-loading equipment such as dumbbells.

- Perform the lift with the correct form and controlled speed.

- Breathe normally during a lift; breathe *out* when the weight is lifted and *in* when the weight is lowered.

- Don't "bounce" weights off your body; use a lighter weight.

- Be in a stable and controlled position prior to the lift.

- Always select a load that is within your capacity to lift.

If you observe any equipment problem that can be a safety hazard, report it at once to the fitness supervisor.

WEIGHT TRAINING

Arm Curl

With arms extended, hold the barbell with an underhand grip. While keeping the elbows close to the sides, flex the forearms and raise the barbell to the chest; lower to the starting position.

Suggested beginning load: 1/4 to 1/3 of body weight

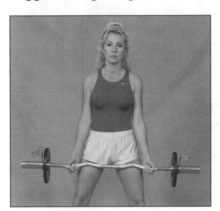 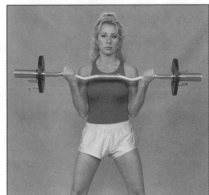

Overhead Press

Hold the barbell at chest level with an overhand grip. Push the bar straight up to full extension and then lower to the starting position. Do not hyperextend the back.

Suggested beginning load: 1/4 to 1/3 of body weight

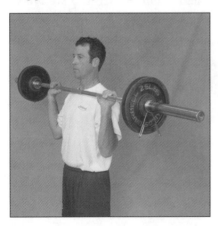 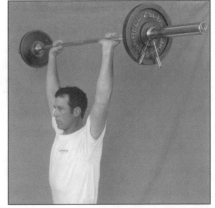

Bench Press

Hold barbell above chest with hands slightly wider than shoulder width. Lower barbell to chest and push back to starting position.

Suggested beginning load: 1/4 to 1/3 of body weight

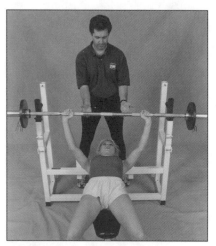
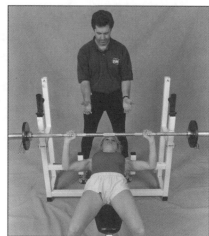

Upright Rowing

Hold barbell with an overhand grip with hands one to two inches apart. Keep elbows above the bar while raising it to shoulder position.

Suggested beginning load: 1/4 to 1/3 of body weight

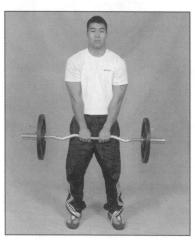
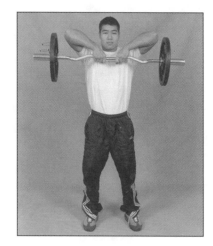

Heel Lifts

With barbell behind shoulder at the back of the neck, raise upward on toes and then slowly return heels to the floor, 10–15 times.

Suggested beginning load: 1/2 to 2/3 of body weight

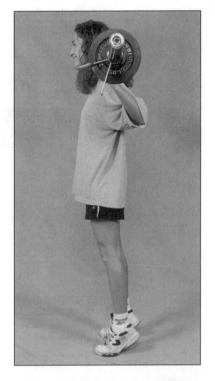

Half-Squats

With barbell behind shoulders at the back of the neck, gradually lower body to a semi-squat position, 10–15 times.

Suggested beginning load: 1/2 to 2/3 of body weight

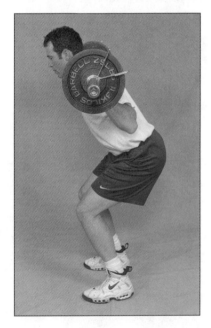

Muscular Strength and Endurance Without Weights

Generally, if your training program includes running, cycling, or dancing, you are providing enough stimulus to maintain an adequate level of muscular strength and endurance in your leg muscles. However, those activities do little for the muscular strength of your arms, shoulders, or trunk. One of the most common exercises to increase muscular strength and endurance for these muscle groups are those in which your own body acts as the weight or resistance against which you work. The activities in the following section focus attention on strength and endurance development in the arms and shoulders.

UPPER BODY

Push-Away

Start developing your upper body with the push-away until you can comfortably do three sets of 10 in one workout.

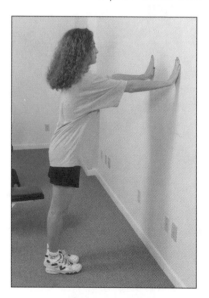 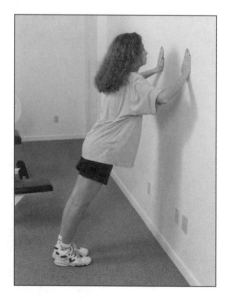

Bent-Knee Push-Up

Once you meet your goal for push-aways, try the bent-knee push-up, starting with two sets of 5 and increasing until you can do two sets of 10 in a single workout.

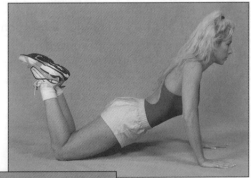

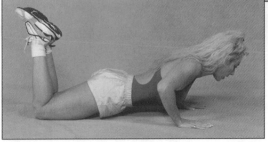

Full-Body Push-Up

Finally, shift to the full-body push-up, doing two sets of 5 and gradually work up to two sets of 10. When you have accomplished this goal, continue to do the two sets of 10 in each workout.

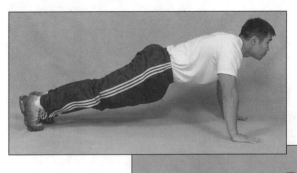

Modified Pull-Up

Body weight is partially supported in the modified pull-up, making it easier to do than the standard pull-up. We recommend that you use a lower bar—when lying on your back, the bar should be a few inches above your outstretched arms. Start with two or three modified pull-ups, adding some when you are able, gradually working up to doing 25 to 35.

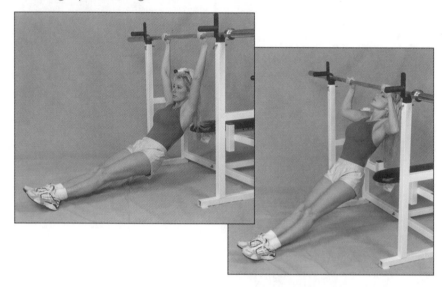

Pull-Up

The standard pull-up is difficult to do because the entire body weight must be pulled up. It is not uncommon for some people to be unable to do a single pull-up.

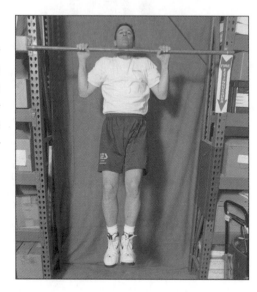

Modified Dip

Another exercise that you can use to strengthen your upper body is the "dip." The modified, weight-supported version is easier to do than the regular dip.

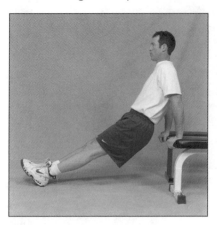
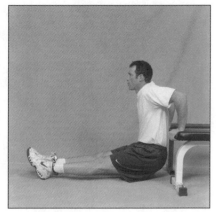

Weight-Bearing Dip

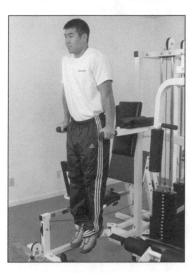
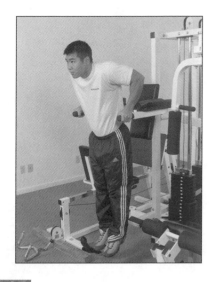

Smart fitness includes muscular strength and endurance exercises. By following the suggestions outlined in this chapter for adding a muscular fitness element to your overall fitness program, you will enhance your bone density and find that physical tasks can be done with ease and confidence.

chapter 8

Staying Injury Free

When you cross the street, drive a car, operate a lawn mower, or climb a ladder, you are risking injury. If even these common tasks have a risk of injury, it should be no surprise that participation in a physical activity program, even one related to improving health status, is not without risks as well.

Injury Risks

Evidence suggests that the risk of injury increases for workouts conducted at intensities greater than 85 percent of maximal heart rate, durations longer than 40 minutes, and frequencies greater than four times per week. Activities such as running and exercising to music cause more muscle and skeletal trauma than riding a stationary cycle or swimming do. Games, especially competitive ones, are associated with more injuries than are controlled, low-intensity, cooperative games.

However, the potential for injury goes beyond the type, intensity, frequency, and duration of activity. The environment and the characteristics of the participant also contribute to overall injury risk. Exercising in a hot, humid environment predisposes one to heat injury, while exercising in the cold can lead to frostbite and hypothermia. Not surprisingly, older, less fit people are more susceptible to skeletal injuries than are young, fit people. Finally, someone with a medical condition such as asthma or diabetes requires special attention to avoid a situation that could result in serious trouble. The purpose of all this is not to scare you to the point of not participating in an exercise program, but rather to address safety issues in order to minimize the risks associated with such programs.

Minimizing Risk of Injury

As we have indicated in preceding chapters, one of the most important things to do to minimize risk is to undergo a health screening before beginning an exercise program. On the basis of the screening you may be referred for additional tests, placed in a medically supervised program, or told that exercising in a graduated program such as the one described in chapter 10 represents a low risk.

Our recommended exercise program suggests starting slowly, progressing in an orderly fashion from low to moderate intensities, and avoiding more uncontrolled activities until you achieve a solid fitness base. It is important to listen to your body, pay attention to signals that indicate you may be doing too much, and slow down if such signals appear. Even if you heed this advice, however, you may still experience an injury during exercise. Therefore we must move beyond these recommendations and discuss the treatment of common injuries associated with exercise.

Common Injuries

One of the most common problems associated with starting an exercise program is muscle soreness. It is important to understand that muscle soreness is normal when beginning any new physical activity.

If you are an avid jogger who puts in 12 miles a week and you decide to participate in a game of soccer, which emphasizes sudden bursts of speed, changes of direction, and explosive kicks, don't be surprised by the muscle soreness that shows up 24 to 48 hours after the game. The soreness is the result of tissue damage in the active muscles and the inflammation response (swelling) that follows. Once you have experienced soreness, it usually does not recur in those muscles as a result of the same activity unless a long period of time (6 to 9 weeks)

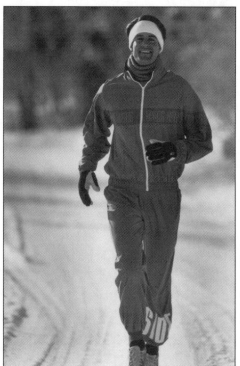

© International Stock/Caroline Wood

PROTECTION FROM THE ENVIRONMENT

- If you are allergic to bee or ant stings get a prescription for an epinephrine auto-injector from your doctor and carry it with you.
- Mosquitoes, flies, lice, fleas, and ticks can be vectors for serious diseases (e.g., plague, encephalitis, malaria, typhus, and Lyme disease). To protect yourself, use insect repellents that contain diethyltoluamide (DEET) or permethrin.
- Do not exercise in an area where motor vehicle traffic is congested, causing an accumulation of carbon monoxide. Keep an eye on air pollution. Daily papers usually give reports on the Pollution Standards Index (PSI) in polluted areas. PSI scores have a range of 0 to 500. A score above 100 is unhealthy.
- Use safe equipment. All equipment (e.g., helmets, scuba gear) must be approved by American National Standards Institute (ANSI) and carry its label.
- Change your running/walking shoes after 500 miles. In addition, give attention to the shoes you wear every day. Many hard, heavy, and pointed shoes (especially high heels) shape our feet in unhealthy ways and can lead to problems. After some use, sneakers may turn upward from the front of their soles, causing involuntary extension of toes and decreasing proper contact with the ground.

Climbing

- If you are going to exercise above 8,000 feet, find out about altitude sickness.
- If your heart beats faster and you are short of breath, stop and descend 2,000 feet. If you are not feeling any better, see your doctor as soon as possible. Symptoms such as confusion, a hacking cough, and having trouble walking indicate the need for immediate medical attention.
- Allow time for your body to adapt to decreasing oxygen levels.
- Take one day to climb each 1,000 feet above 8,000 feet.
- Limit your alcohol intake and drink a lot of water. In general, diet or vitamins do not help altitude sickness.

How to Prevent Being Struck by Lightning

- Estimate the distance of the storm: every five seconds between the flash and the sound of thunder equals one mile.
- Do not stand on high, open fields or under an isolated tree.
- Descend to below timberline from mountain peaks.

- Do not stay in water, which is an excellent conductor.
- Get to a safe place or your car and close doors and windows.
- Keep away from metal objects or sport gear.
- If you are caught in an open area, go to a low place and stay in a curled position, tucking your feet under your body.

Ultraviolet (UV) Light/Sunlight

- Skin cancer is the most common type of cancer and exposure to UV/sunlight is the most common cause. Research tells us that its development is not consistent with duration of exposure: a few strong exposures can trigger it. However, early diagnosis can be lifesaving. Examine your skin thoroughly in front of a mirror. Watch for moles and spots with the following characteristics: asymmetry and irregular borders, loss of color uniformity, a diameter greater than a pencil tip, and elevation from the surrounding skin.
- Watch for medicines that interact with sunlight and cause adverse effects (e.g., tetracycline).
- Always use sunscreens that provide a skin protection factor (SPF) greater than 15. Apply them generously to all areas that will be exposed to the sun, including your lips, before you go out. Reapply sunscreens after excessive sweating or swimming.
- Wear a hat with a brim three to four inches wide.
- Protect your skin even on cloudy days and when you are in the shade. UV light is well reflected to your skin from sand, water, cement, and snow.
- Sunlight is strongest between 10 A.M. and 3 P.M. and much stronger at high altitudes.
- Keep away from tanning parlors, which expose your skin to extreme doses of UV.
- Synthetic tan lotions do not protect from UV.
- Any suntan means skin damage. Repeated damage will wrinkle your skin and can cause cancer.

Prevention of Exercise-Induced Asthma

- Do not exercise in cold and polluted air. Warm and humid air is best.
- Take your medicines and warm up before exercise.
- Avoid intense and continuous exertion such as jogging. Try sports with short bursts of exertion (e.g., football, soccer, baseball, tennis).
- Breathe through your nose and do not hyperventilate.

elapses between exposures. The following signs and symptoms associated with injury are listed to call your attention to circumstances that may require special attention:

- Extreme tenderness when body part is touched
- Pain while at rest, pain that will not disappear after warming up, joint pain, increased pain when moving or exercising that body part
- Swelling or discoloration
- Changes in normal body function

Though these signs and symptoms can also appear in an extreme case of muscle soreness, in general they do not. We encourage you to discuss them with your fitness instructor and physician.

Treatment for Common Injuries

The most common injuries associated with exercise programs are sprains and strains. Sprains are caused by the stretching of the connective tissue (ligaments) surrounding a joint, while strains occur when muscles or tendons are stretched. The immediate treatment of both conditions is summed up by the acronym *PRICE*, which stands for *Protecting* and *Resting* the injured body part, using *Ice* with *Compression*, and *Elevating* it to reduce fluid accumulation.

The following steps will help to reduce the swelling associated with an injury and reduce the time needed for normal function to return. Follow these same steps when a muscle is damaged by a direct blow (contusion) or when the heel of the foot strikes a hard surface causing a "stone bruise." In the case of a contusion the muscle should usually be stretched before the ice is applied, and for a heel bruise a soft pad should be placed under the heel to reduce the force of impact.

- *Protect* the body part from further damage.
- *Rest* the body part: do not try to "walk it off."
- *Ice* helps to reduce the blood flow to the injured site as well as the sensation of pain. Apply ice (crushed or cubes in a plastic bag) for 20 to 30 minutes and repeat on a regular basis—hourly or when pain occurs. Ice treatment should continue for 24 to 72 hours depending on the degree of injury.

- *Compression* bandages should be used to hold the ice bag in place and also when the ice is removed. The bandage should be wrapped firmly, but not too tightly, to help minimize swelling.
- *Elevate* the injured body part whenever possible.

Moderate injuries (exhibiting swelling, discoloration, and joint tenderness) to severe injuries (exhibiting extreme tenderness and swelling, discoloration, and deformity of the body part) should be examined by a physician. Always remember to follow the PRICE steps for any acute (recent) injury. You may apply heat later in the recovery process when the swelling and the chance of more bleeding (which causes more swelling) are reduced. In addition, people with chronic problems such as tendonitis or bursitis may apply heat *prior to* the activity. If you are ever in doubt, use ice.

Common Orthopedic Problems

Orthopedic problems may relate to skeletal muscles, connective tissue (both tendons and ligaments), or tissues in or around joints. While infection and direct physical trauma can cause many orthopedic problems, overuse is the most common cause. Following is a brief list of common conditions:

- *Bursitis*—Inflammation of the bursa, which is a fluid-filled sac between muscle and bone that aids in movement
- *Tendonitis*—Inflammation of a tendon, which is the tissue tying a muscle to a bone
- *Myositis*—Inflammation of a muscle
- *Synovitis*—Inflammation of the synovial membrane, which forms the inner lining of joint cavities and secretes synovial fluid to aid in the movement of the bones in the joint space
- *Plantar Fasciitis*—Inflammation of the connective tissue on the bottom of the foot

The constant in all of these conditions is inflammation, which is the body's normal reaction to infection or trauma. Inflammation involves special white blood cells as well as chemicals that expand the pores in capillaries to let large proteins enter the injured area. This influx of protein brings water along, causing the swelling. Tennis elbow and shin splints (more on these later) are examples of inflammatory reactions involving muscles and connective tissue.

Overuse Problems

The immediate treatment for these problems is the same as for sprains: ice and rest. If the problem is a chronic (long-term) one, warming the area before physical activity and using ice afterward can help reduce pain and discomfort. An obvious recommendation is to stop doing the activity that causes the problem and shift to another activity. For joggers who develop problems with their knees, swimming is a good substitute. For swimmers who develop shoulder problems, cycling is a good substitute. If any chronic inflammatory condition limits your normal daily function, see your physician.

Stress fractures to the lower leg and the foot are also caused by overuse. This problem occurs when the bone's ability to adapt to a chronic load is exceeded. The area over the fracture is very tender to the touch. Pain is present most of the time but increases when you stand. Stress fractures need a physician's care and take a long time to heal (6 to 10 weeks). Any supplemental exercises you use during the recovery process must be approved by your physician.

Shin Splints

Shin splints refer to an inflammation of the muscle-tendon unit on the front side of the lower leg. This injury has a wide variety of causes, including overuse. It is more common in runners and dancers (including participants in exercise-to-music programs) because of the special load these participants place on the lower leg during exercise. However, weak arches, hard surfaces, inadequate shoes, structural abnormalities, and improper exercise techniques can all cause shin splints. Needless to say, the recommended ways to deal with this injury are as varied as the list of causes.

- *Overuse*—Cut back on the total amount of running or dancing, or simply substitute something else.
- *Surface*—Running or dancing on softer surfaces will help absorb the shock of impact.

- *Shoes*—Well-cushioned and properly designed exercise shoes will help to dissipate the shock of impact.

Don't be fooled into believing that the simple purchase of an excellent (and expensive!) pair of exercise shoes will make shin splints disappear. Shoes can help reduce the problem, but you must also exercise good judgment about the overuse issue. Some people use their good shoes and soft floor as a rationale to exercise even more, resulting in an aggravation of the problem. Add variety to your workout to reduce the chance that you will overstress any single area of your body.

Heat Injuries

The following signs and symptoms may indicate trouble:

- Hair standing on end on arms, back, and chest
- Chills
- Throbbing in the head, or headache
- Vomiting or nausea
- Dry lips or "cotton mouth"
- Muscle cramping
- Light-headedness
- No sweating

The following is a set of guidelines regarding exercise in heat and humidity:

- When very hot, humid weather is forecast, exercise in the cooler part of the day.
- Gradually increase your exposure to the heat and humidity over a period of 7 to 10 days.
- Wear clothing that facilitates the evaporation of sweat.
- Reduce the intensity of the exercise.
- Drink extra water before exercise, drink during exercise, and replace what you have lost after exercise.
- If you must, use additional salt at mealtime. Do not take salt tablets.
- If you feel light-headed, nauseated, or flushed, stop exercising; get out of the heat; drink water; and cool down with wet cloths, fans, and so forth.

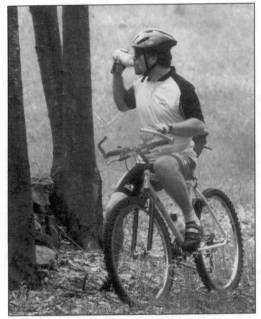

© Terry Wild Studio

Modification of Exercise for Safety

Table 8.1 classifies injuries as *mild*, *moderate*, and *severe* and offers some suggestions on how to deal with them. This list is not a prescription to follow. If you hear a "pop," feel a deformity, or think you have a serious injury, contact a physician.

For those injuries you believe to be mild, we suggest you find activities that minimize the role of the injured part. Often you can use water or cycling (with legs or arms) exercises that do not affect the injury. In some cases, you may have to refrain from your usual exercise until the injury is better.

EXERCISE IN THE COLD

- Do not exercise in extreme cold and wind; use indoor activities.
- Wear layers of clothing, removing them one at a time as you warm up.
- Stay as dry as possible.

Table 8.1

Injury Classification Criteria and Exercise Modifications

Criteria	Modifications
Mild injury	
Performance is not affected. Pain is experienced only after athletic activity. Generally, no tenderness is felt on palpation. No or minimal swelling is present. No discoloration is apparent.	Reduce activity level, modify activity to take stress off the injured part, treat symptomatically, and gradually return to full activity.
Moderate injury	
Performance is mildly affected or not affected at all. Pain is experienced before and after athletic activity. Mild tenderness is felt on palpation. Mild swelling may be present. Some discoloration may be present.	Rest the injured part, modify activity to take stress off the injured part, treat symptomatically, and gradually return to full activity.
Severe injury	
Pain is experienced before, during, and after activity. Performance is definitely affected because of pain. Normal daily function is affected because of pain. Movement is limited because of pain. Moderate to severe point tenderness is felt on palpation. Swelling is most likely present. Discoloration may be present.	Rest completely and see a physician.

Reprinted, by permission, from E.T. Howley and B.D. Franks, 1997, *Health Fitness Instructor's Handbook*, 3d ed. (Champaign, IL: Human Kinetics), 429.

If your own exercise modifications do not result in a relief of the problem after two to four weeks, consult a physician. When the injured part gets better, do very light exercises involving that part and gradually increase the intensity. Avoid quick movements of the injured part. Trying to do too much too soon after an injury often results in reinjury.

Any activity we undertake can be risky, and a fitness program is no exception. However, by following the suggestions outlined in this chapter, with a healthy dose of common sense thrown in, you can reduce your risk of injury as you begin your fitness program.

chapter 9

Coping With Stress

Physical fitness encompasses many aspects of our physical selves, including cardiovascular function, relative leanness, low back function, muscular strength and endurance, and flexibility. Though we acknowledge our inability to separate the mental, physical, psychological, social, and spiritual aspects of life, this book emphasizes physical fitness. In this chapter we address an area that bridges the psychological and physiological aspects of fitness.

Psychological Aspects of Fitness

The healthy person can work and play with vigor and enthusiasm and is able to relax and disregard irrelevant stimuli during quiet times. Vitality and relaxation are both enhanced by physical conditioning. One of the keys to living the healthy life is balancing arousal and relaxation. People who are always relaxed and easygoing don't accomplish very much. On the other hand, people who have a "get up and go" attitude toward all aspects of life exhibit coronary-prone behavior.

This chapter deals with the idea of balance by describing the relationships among personality, physical activity, stress, and health. It is beyond the scope of the chapter to discuss extensively all psychological aspects of fitness. Our concern here is with "normal" levels of personality and stress and their implications for fitness programs.

Personality and Physical Activity

Because individuals perceive and react to the same situation differently, it is impossible to predict exactly how a person will respond psychologically and physiologically to a specific external stimulus. One movie may evoke anger, laughter, and no emotion in three different people. Playing a game in front of a crowd might cause best or worst performances in different players. Part of the reason people differ in their perceptions and reactions is related to personality.

Types A and B

Authorities agree that personality and the ability to cope with stress are related to coronary heart disease (CHD). However, the exact characteristics that cause the higher risk are difficult to enumerate or measure. One attempt to do this separates people into Type A and Type B behavior. People with Type A behavior (extremely time conscious, angry, aggressive, impatient) are more prone to CHD. If you exhibit these characteristics, then you have a greater response to psychological stressors. Therefore, it is appropriate to learn to relax, be cautious about overdoing exercise, and be engaged in more relatively noncompetitive activities. If, on the other hand, you are a Type B person (easygoing, nonaggressive, "laid-back"), you may need more stimulation and motivation to begin and continue an exercise program.

Anger

Evidence points to a relationship between anger and CHD. If you keep anger bottled up inside rather than expressing it (e.g., talking about it to a close friend), you are at increased risk for CHD. Three recommendations can help you with your anger:

1. Try to develop positive attitudes toward yourself, others, and the world in general so that anger occurs less frequently.
2. Express anger rather than denying it or keeping it inside.
3. Develop the kind of relationships with others that allows emotions to be shared.

When you are open about your own feelings ("What you did really made me angry yesterday") and sensitive to other peoples' moods ("You seem upset today"), you are dealing appropriately with anger.

Assertiveness, Aggression, Hostility, and Denial

Assertiveness, aggression, hostility, and denial may, for different reasons, cause you to do too much. If you tend to be an aggressive or hostile person, you may get so involved in your exercise activity that you don't pay attention to discomfort or danger signs. If you try to deny your pain, you tend to overdo. One of the distinctions between assertiveness and aggression or hostility is that the assertive person is sensitive to others, whereas the aggressive or hostile person is less concerned with others' feelings. If you tend to be aggressive, consider the feelings of others in the group. One way of doing this is to ask yourself how you would feel if someone else in the group did to you what you are doing to others.

Anxiety, Depression, and Fear

We all experience some level of anxiety, depression, and fear. Postcardiac patients and other people with low fitness levels, however, often experience high levels of these conditions. If you are unduly worried or afraid about increasing or changing your physical activity, ask for support from the fitness leader. It is important to ease into a fitness program and to see that positive results can occur with minimum risk as you progress to higher levels of activity. Another aspect of becoming physically active and adopting other healthy behaviors is the increased perception of control over your own life, which can help you deal with your anxiety, fear, or depression.

Rationalization

One of the most difficult skills is being able to differentiate between the real reasons for our behavior and the rationalizations we choose to believe. It is impossible to progress with exercise or other healthy behaviors until we acknowledge the real reasons for our current behaviors. Being completely honest with ourselves and the fitness leader is an important step in increasing healthy behaviors.

Rejection

You may have rejected exercise in the past or feel that active persons have rejected you (e.g., as a child you were always the last chosen to play games). Keep in mind when choosing a fitness program that a good program will help everyone feel included and welcome.

Catharsis

Some people use exercise to cleanse their minds and emotions. Their fitness activities relieve the clutter in their minds and allow them to start fresh following the exercise. After you reach a minimum level of fitness, there is a place in the fitness program for activities that allow you to "let go." For example, a runner might include some speed work, sprinting during some sections of the run. Those who play sports for fitness might engage in a vigorous singles match of racquetball, tennis, or one-on-one basketball.

Euphoria

Some people experience a heightened emotional state (sometimes referred to as a "runner's high") while exercising. This state resembles

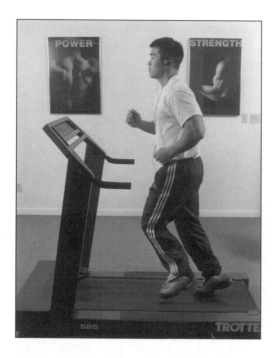

a deep religious experience or the emotional state achieved by using certain drugs. It cannot be planned, nor can it serve as the basis for motivation, since you may not experience it. However, almost everyone can achieve an increased sense of "feeling good" as a result of appropriate physical activities.

One of the main purposes of a fitness program is to help you progress safely to the fitness level at which you become "addicted" in that you look forward to your regular workout. As with all healthy behaviors, however, it is possible to take an exercise addiction to the extreme. Instead of regarding exercise as a healthy part of life, some people become obsessed and overemphasize its importance, spending time exercising instead of spending time in other parts of their lives (e.g., working or with their families).

Motivation

There are two levels of motivation regarding exercise: what will get us to begin a fitness program and what will motivate us to make exercise a regular part of our lives. While we all know in general what healthy behaviors are (most people agree that they should exercise on a regular basis), what will motivate us to begin our own fitness program? Convenient programs that provide personal contact with concerned exercise professionals complement the information we all have about the healthy life and can help us in starting a fitness regime.

Continuing an exercise regime and making it a part of our everyday routines is sometimes more challenging than beginning one. Individual attention, realistic goals with periodic evaluation, an option for group participation, involvement of a spouse and/or important others, contracts, and programs that minimize injury all seem to help people adhere to fitness programs. Fitness has to achieve priority status (like eating and sleeping) in our lives. Any efforts to increase motivation must have that end in sight. Therefore, external, or extrinsic, rewards must be viewed as a temporary means to change behavior—behavior can only be maintained over the long haul with internal, or intrinsic, motivation.

Play and Goal Orientation

One of the key elements in achieving an arousal/relaxation equilibrium and minimizing stress is to appreciate the balance of work and play. One individual may have difficulty taking time just to play and enjoy an activity not directly related to productivity, while another may have a problem in getting down to business and getting a task done. People who try to pattern their fitness programs after military or athletic models often have a goal orientation without the concept of play. Others who are not discriminating about their selection of activities as long as everyone is having a good time may achieve playfulness without fitness gains. The successful fitness program achieves both by including activities designed to improve the necessary fitness components while maintaining a playful atmosphere.

State/Trait

Making the distinction between your "usual" (*trait*) personality characteristics and specific "situational" (*state*) personality characteristics is helpful in dealing with your personality. For example, you may normally be very quiet and introverted but become an extrovert during competitive games. You may normally be very relaxed but may get anxious about exercise. Generally, personality traits do not change very much, or very quickly. Personality and emotional states vary

Exercises for Office Workers

Every hour try to do some of the following exercises:

1. Get up and walk as often and as much as possible.
2. Holding onto the back of a nonrolling chair, squat several times.
3. Holding onto your desk, do partial push-ups several times.
4. Hold your hips with both hands and stretch your trunk slightly backward several times.
5. Bend forward while sitting, drop your arms and head between your knees toward the floor.
6. Sit erect on your chair. Bend your neck forward and to the sides.

with situations and are more susceptible to change. For example, if you are afraid or anxious about a physical activity, try easing into the activity and progressing in small increments until you are relaxed and unafraid when exercising.

Stress Continuums

There is no uniform agreement on what defines stress. Your perception of a stimulus or situation determines to a large extent how stressful it is to you. For our purposes, a stressor is defined as any stimulus or condition that causes physiological arousal beyond what is necessary to accomplish a given activity. This excessive arousal is called stress.

The three major components of stress are the amount by which the stress response exceeds the functional demand, how pleasant it is to the individual, and whether it causes development or deterioration. These components are explained in the following sections.

Functional Versus Severe Stress

An individual's physiological response to stress at any one time lies on a continuum from what is essential to provide the energy for that task to an extreme physiological response beyond what is needed. Table 9.1 illustrates the heart rate necessary to perform various tasks and the additional heart-rate response caused by chronic stressors (e.g., excess fat) and acute stressors (e.g., an agitated emotional state).

Table 9.1

Stress Components of Heart Rate

	HEART RATE, BEATS/MIN		
Component of heart rate	Sitting	Climbing stairs	Running
HR needed to do task	30	50	100
Additional HR due to chronic stressors			
Poor aerobic fitness	+15	+20	+40
Excess fat	+5	+15	+20
Additional HR due to acute stressors			
Not relaxed	+10	+5	0
Emotional state	+15	+10	0
Total heart rate	75	100	160

Note. The actual HR values will vary with the individual depending on body size, fitness level, and type and severity of stressors.
Reprinted, by permission, from E.T. Howley and B.D. Franks, 1997, *Health Fitness Instructor's Handbook*, 3d ed. (Champaign, IL: Human Kinetics), 382.

Enjoyable Versus Unpleasant

Another aspect of stress is how enjoyable you perceive the stressor to be. Attending an exciting concert and taking an examination to qualify for a position may both provoke stress responses; however, most people would probably perceive the concert as more enjoyable.

Development Versus Deterioration

The end result of stress is somewhat independent of the other two aspects of stress. For example, a stressful event (i.e., one that causes a large stress response beyond what is essential physically) can result in your being inspired to achieve great things, or it may destroy your initiative. On the other hand, conditions that cause little stress response may lead to steady development or can gradually wear down your desire to excel. In addition, you can grow and develop from stressors that are pleasant (e.g., positive reinforcement) as well as those that are unpleasant (e.g., a deadline to finish a project).

It is important to realize that either pleasant or unpleasant stressors may keep you from confronting important areas of your life. Be cautious about identifying a specific stressor as healthy or unhealthy based only on the degree of physiological and psychological stress response or how pleasant you find the situation. A better criterion is whether the experience has led you toward higher levels of mental, social, and/or physical health.

Relationship of Stress to Health

Stress affects health both positively and negatively. No discussion of the highest quality of life possible nor of serious health problems is complete without including the issue of stress.

Positive Stress

We often think of stress as a primarily negative influence on our lives, but it has many positive features, including the following:

- *Variety*—Stimuli and stressors are important components of the full life. You would live a bland existence without stress.
- *Development and Growth*—We cannot develop, learn, grow, and strive toward our optimal potential without encountering stress.
- *Special High Moments*—One feature of the good life is special emotional experiences that are remembered forever. It is likely that these peak moments were stressful.

Negative Stress

The issue of stress must be included in any discussion of our society's health problems.

Secondary Risk Factor

Stress is listed as a risk factor for many major health problems—coronary heart disease, hypertension, cancer, ulcers, low back pain, and headaches, for example. Although an inability to cope with stress is probably insufficient by itself to cause any of these problems, stress does seem to exacerbate them. In some people, stress results in a heart attack; in others, it results in hypertension, ulcers, low back pain, or headaches.

Susceptibility to Other Stressors

While it is unclear whether coping well with one stressor helps us in coping with others, there is little doubt that coping poorly with one stressor hampers our ability to cope with others. All of us have found ourselves getting upset (stressed) over something that normally would not bother us because of stressors in other areas of our lives. Two aspects of our inability to cope are our perceptions of and reactions to stressors.

Physical Activity and Stress Reduction

Many writers have justified exercise programs partly on the basis that they reduce stress. Although the claims have often exceeded the evidence, there is some support for the assertion that stress is reduced as a result of a single period or bout of exercise (acute exercise) as well as over the course of a conditioning program (chronic exercise). Too much exercise, however, can be an additional stressor for people at all levels of fitness. The following illustrations of how exercise can reduce stress assume that you exercise enough but not too much.

Acute Activity

Single bouts of exercise can reduce stress in three primary ways.

• *Distraction*—Exercise (like many other activities) can serve as a temporary distraction from stressors. It is often helpful to step away from a problem, then come back to it later. This technique is healthful as long as exercise doesn't become an escape from the problem. Ultimately, stress can be reduced only by coping with the stressor(s). However, one part of your coping strategy can be the distraction of physical activity. Learn to "listen" to your body's signals as to when is a good time to step away from a problem and do a fitness workout.

• *Control of Situations*—A perception of personal control can strengthen our ability to cope with stressors. In some cases exercise enhances this feeling of control. For example, increased practice and skill acquisition as a result of an exercise program can result in reduced stress when playing a game in the presence of others. One of the benefits of a postcardiac exercise program is that it reduces the participant's fear that any exertion will cause another heart attack, thus increasing the participant's feelings of control over his or her life.

• *Interaction With Others*—A third way that acute exercise may influence stress is by offering solitude. For some people one of their daily stressors is constant contact with other people. For example, a working parent spends almost every waking moment in the presence of others—children, spouse, employees, employer, colleagues—who demand time and attention. That person can use a walking or jogging program as time to be alone with his or her thoughts. At the other extreme is a person who has little contact with others during a typical day, with loneliness being a potential stressor. In this case, participating with other people in an exercise program can be helpful.

Chronic Activity

A regular exercise program can also result in stress reduction over the long term.

• *Reduction of Chronic Stressors*—Increased cardiorespiratory function and decreased body fat cause you to be less stressed throughout the day.

• *Reduction of Exercise Stress*—With increased fitness levels, physical activity itself becomes less of a stressor. Numerous studies have shown that as a person becomes fit, he or she can do the same amount of external work with a lower heart rate, lower blood pressure, and reduced adrenaline production. Thus the functional response to the work (the energy necessary to accomplish the task) remains the same, but the stress response is reduced.

• *Adaptation to Other Stressors*—Increased adaptation to exercise may carry over to adaptation to other stressors, although this theory has inconsistent support. Some believe, with some evidence, that adaptation to physical activity provides a basis for better adaptation to other stressors. Others believe, also with some evidence, that adaptation is specific to given stimuli and stressors. This question needs additional research.

Coping With Stress

People can do many things to maximize the positive aspects of stress while minimizing the negative aspects. Being involved in a variety of different situations, improving coping skills, and increasing control of one's life are some of the elements of a healthy lifestyle related to stress.

Exposure to Many Stressors

Simply being exposed to a wide range of experiences helps you become better educated and less stressed by new situations. A good fitness program provides a variety of different types of experiences, including cooperative, problem-solving, competitive, individual, partner, and team activities. This variety helps by improving fitness while also increasing the ability to cope with different movement experiences.

Increasing Coping Abilities

People use many different strategies in dealing with stress. Facing the problem, looking at alternatives, talking about it with close friends, seeking professional or technical advice, and stepping back or away from the problem for a brief time are all behaviors people use in coping with stress. Which ones are better suited for particular situations? Are there some you think might help but that you feel uncomfortable trying? You can begin to practice coping behaviors in "easy" settings. In terms of fitness, the variety of activities in a good program require different coping strategies. For example, different coping skills are required in cooperative and competitive activities, as well as in those done alone or with others.

Development of Optimal Fitness

Becoming more fit physically, mentally, and socially will cause potential stressors to be less threatening. If you can do hard work, then you do not dread physical stressors. If you are accustomed to the mental processes that lead to problem solving, then having a difficult problem is not as stressful. Establishing meaningful relationships with other people can assist you in having positive responses to stressful social situations.

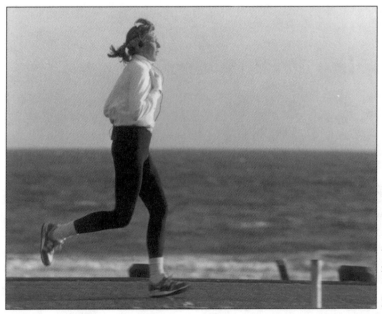

© Terry Wild Studio

Control

Authorities repeatedly list perception of control as a major element in coping with stress. Therefore, whatever you can do to help gain control of your life will diminish the negative effects of potentially stressful conditions.

Healthy Behaviors

One of the by-products of exercising, eating nutritious foods, and refraining from using harmful drugs is the feeling that you are taking responsibility for your own life. Not only do the healthy behaviors themselves reduce stress, but the fact that you have "taken charge" also reduces stress levels. Chapter 2 includes recommendations about ways to increase healthy behaviors.

Competence

Give attention to whatever activities, tasks, and relationships are important to you so that you can increase your skills in those areas. Your self-confidence will increase as you experience greater success with the things that matter most to you.

Assertiveness

It is also important to recognize when unreasonable demands are being made of you, whether by you or by someone else. It is essential to good health to be able to point out the problem and work with others (e.g., your boss or your spouse) to accomplish common goals in a reasonable way within an appropriate time frame.

Relaxation

Knowing how to relax is an important aspect of overall health. Many relaxation techniques have been developed, including the "relaxation response" technique by Benson and colleagues. One easily used technique (described below), introduced by Edmund Jacobson in 1938, aims at helping you recognize the feelings produced by tension.

Begin by getting in a comfortable position with eyes closed. It is recommended that you lie down, but it can be done in a sitting position as well. Tense a specific area of the body (e.g., your foot), hold for about 20 seconds, then relax; then tense a larger segment (e.g., your leg), hold, relax, and so on. Feel the tension while holding, then feel the tension leave the area during the period of relaxation. The following sequence can be used:

- Right toes
- Left toes
- Right foot
- Left foot
- Right leg below knee
- Left leg below knee
- Right leg below hip
- Left leg below hip
- Both legs below hips
- Abdomen and buttocks
- Right fingers
- Left fingers
- Right arm below elbow
- Left arm below elbow
- Right arm below shoulder
- Left arm below shoulder
- Both arms below shoulders
- Chest
- Neck
- Jaw
- Forehead
- Entire head
- Entire body

Extend the last relaxation period and feel the tension leaving your body. Now lie still and consciously experience your breathing.

Stress is a part of all of our lives. While excessive stress can be debilitating and can even compromise our health, many forms of stress are beneficial. By maximizing the positive elements of stress, developing a range of coping abilities, exhibiting healthy behaviors, and gaining as much control as possible over our lives, we are better able to deal with the inevitable conditions of stress. Coping with stress, and growing from it, should be part of every fitness program.

chapter **10**

Designing
a Complete
Fitness Program

Chapters 5 through 7 addressed the various components of fitness. This chapter begins with the two basic principles introduced briefly in chapter 7: *overload* and *specificity*.

Principles of a Fitness Program

In order for any body tissue to increase in function it must be exposed to a load greater than that to which it is accustomed; the tissue then gradually adapts to this load by increasing its size or function. The process of overload followed by adaptation is the basis of fitness and performance programs and is called the *principle of overload*. An example of this principle is a person whose heart function is weak due to years of sedentary living. Such a person can overload the heart and the entire cardiorespiratory system simply by slow walking. Gradually, the heart gets stronger, and the person has to walk faster to overload the heart. After several months of working up to fast walking for several miles, the heart becomes strong enough to handle the walking easily. Any further improvement in cardiorespiratory function requires that the person jog or racewalk. Exercise intensity must be increased gradually, and adaptation must be evident before a move is made to a higher intensity.

The process also works in the opposite direction—if an individual stops working against that load, the system returns to its former "untrained" state. This is sometimes referred to as the principle of reversibility. In short, the old adage "use it or lose it" is true.

The second major principle of training is *specificity*, which means that the type of adaptation that occurs is related to the type of exercise. For example, different adaptations would occur if one identical twin participated in cardiovascular endurance exercises while his brother participated in a weight training program. The first twin would have a leaner body (less fat), better heart function, and muscles with an increased capacity to work without fatigue. The other twin would show an increase in muscle mass and strength with little change in heart function. In each case the muscles were "overloaded," but the type of load was different—endurance activity for one and resistive work for the other. Muscles respond to these unique overloads by adapting in specific ways.

Aspects of a Fitness Program

After you have made some basic decisions about a fitness program based on your health status (see chapter 1), you need to consider some general questions and recommendations in a logical sequence. In general, a fitness program should strive to achieve the goals outlined in chapter 3 and chapters 5 through 7.

Screening

Determining your health status is an important first step in becoming fit. Appendix A includes a health status questionnaire to help you judge whether it is appropriate for you to begin an exercise program. If you have not already done so, go to Appendix A and fill out the questionnaire.

Regular Physical Activity

Once you have determined that you are capable of participating in a fitness program, you must make a commitment to regular physical activity *before* you begin the program. Improvements in fitness levels are both lost and gained quickly. The only way to maintain the fitness levels you achieve is to participate in a regular program of physical activity. In addition, if exercise is to be useful in a weight-control program, it must be done on a regular basis. Just look at former champion athletes who now lead sedentary lives; you will see that neither fitness nor desirable body composition lasts long once activity ends.

Start Slowly

For many people it has been several years since they were active and fit. If it took years for you to get out of shape, it is reasonable that you should allow three to five months or so to get into shape. You will find that it does not take a great deal of activity initially to "overload" the body and create a training effect. For that reason, and because you wish to minimize the likelihood of sore muscles and injury, you should begin an exercise program slowly. It is better to do too little than too much. Although the idea of "no pain, no gain" may be appropriate to athletes training for championship competition, it is irresponsible when applied to fitness programs.

Do too little rather than too much at the start of your fitness program.

Warm-Up and Cool-Down

Just as it is important for you to gradually build up from light work to moderate work over a period of weeks and months, it is also important to include a progression in each workout. Begin each exercise session with some low-intensity activities, including some appropriate stretching and strengthening exercises (see chapters 6 and 7). The warm-up provides a smooth transition from the resting state to the higher level of energy expenditure and effort in the main part of your workout.

At the end of the exercise session, gradually diminish the intensity to allow your body to make the transition back to rest. This will reduce your chances of experiencing light-headedness, which can sometimes occur when you stop an activity suddenly. The cool-down can include some of the same stretches used in the warm-up to further stretch the muscles when they are warm. If an exercise session must be shortened due to lack of time, keep the warm-up and cool-down periods and reduce the time you spend in the main part of your workout.

Periodic Testing

One of the major differences between fitness programs offered by health and fitness professionals and other fitness programs is the opportunity for self-evaluation. A good fitness program provides periodic testing of the various fitness components to give you feedback about how you are doing in relation to your goals.

A general rule of thumb is to make about a 10 percent change over a three-month period in the areas that need improvement. Once you achieve your goal, periodic testing provides evidence that you are holding your own. If you are doing your fitness program on your own, use the various self-tests for each fitness component that we have provided in chapters 5 through 7. You might want to test yourself at three months, six months, one year, and then annually to determine your progress.

Frequency of Workouts

Both light to moderate and vigorous activity should be part of your regular fitness regime. After including light to moderate activity in your regular routine each day, we recommend adding additional moderate to vigorous exercise to achieve both cardiovascular fitness and weight-loss goals three or four times per week—or about every other day. (The same recommendation holds for muscular strength and endurance training programs.) Exercising fewer than three times a week requires a very high intensity of activity to achieve a cardiovascular training effect, and the higher intensity is associated with more injuries. In addition, it is difficult to achieve a weight-loss goal when you exercise fewer than three times a week. If you exercise strenuously more than four times a week, the risk of injury increases. A daily light to moderate routine combined with a day-on, day-off routine for more vigorous activity seems to be optimal and makes an exercise program easy to schedule.

Total Energy Cost and Length of Each Workout

Spending at least 30 minutes in light to moderate activity daily, plus expending 200 to 300 calories per exercise session every other day is recommended in order to achieve a cardiovascular training effect and meet body composition goals. The total caloric cost of a workout is determined by the duration and intensity of the workout (see chapter 5). Generally, you need about 30 to 40 minutes during a workout to achieve a 200- to 300-calorie expenditure when working at the appropriate intensity, since some time is spent in flexibility and warm-up activities. If you do very light activity, then the duration has to be extended in order to achieve the caloric-expenditure goal.

Progression

The first step in beginning a fitness program is to include more activity as part of daily living (e.g., walking instead of driving when possible). The second step is to accumulate at least 30 minutes of

Participate in daily light to moderate physical activity plus vigorous exercise three to four times a week on a day-on, day-off basis.

moderate-intensity activity daily. You should be able to walk four miles briskly before undertaking more strenuous activity. By achieving this goal, you will have established a regular pattern of activity and made some body composition changes that will make the transition to more strenuous exercise easier. After you are able to jog 3 miles (or walk 6 miles briskly, cycle 12 miles, or swim 3/4 of a mile), then you may want to include some games and sports as part of your fitness program. The progression from walking to jogging to running should occur over a period of months.

Intensity

When you are at the stage of incorporating at least 30 minutes of light to moderate activity into your daily routine, there is no need to emphasize doing the activity at a certain intensity level. When you have progressed to including more vigorous activity on alternate days, then you are ready to consider the issue of exercise intensity.

Exercise intensity is best described by the overload it places on the cardiorespiratory system during a workout. The *threshold* needed to achieve the training effect is lower for the very sedentary (50 percent of maximal cardiorespiratory function) compared to the very fit (85 percent of maximal cardiorespiratory function). The primary way to judge exercise intensity is to see how high your heart rate is during the activity, since heart rate increases in a regular manner with exercise intensity. You can estimate your appropriate exercise intensity by calculating a *target heart rate (THR) zone*. The THR zone represents the range of heart-rate values that are high enough to cause a training effect yet low enough to allow you to exercise long enough to achieve the total work needed for a training effect.

As you will see from the following example, the 50-year-old does not have to exercise at a very high heart rate to achieve a training effect. This is a central point in beginning a fitness program. Begin at the low end of the THR zone and be more concerned about doing long-duration, low-intensity exercise than the opposite. Furthermore, we strongly recommend that participants be able to walk four miles

- Daily light to moderate physical activity for at least 30 minutes.
- Vigorous exercise every other day for long enough to expend about 200 to 300 calories.

CALCULATING THR

The first step in calculating THR is to estimate your maximal heart rate. Complete the following:

220 – age (years) = age-adjusted maximal heart rate

Example: For a 50-year-old person, 220 – 50 = 170 beats per minute

Now use your own age: 220 – _____ (years) = _____ beats per minute

The second step is to calculate the THR zone:

70 percent maximal heart rate = low end of THR zone

Example: 70 percent of 170 beats per minute = 119 beats per minute

For you, .70 · _____ beats per minute = _____ beats per minute

85 percent maximal heart rate = high end of THR zone

Example: 85 percent of 170 beats per minute = 145 beats per minute

For you: .85 · _____ beats per minute = _____ beats per minute

before they become concerned about exercise intensity. Many individuals may be able to reach their THR with walking exercise alone.

Although some electronic devices can give you your heart rate "on the go," they are not necessary. If you monitor your heart rate immediately after stopping exercise, the value is a good estimate of what your heart rate was during the exercise. Within 5 seconds after stopping the exercise, count the pulse rate at your neck or wrist for 10 seconds. Since heart rate decreases quickly after exercise is stopped, you must monitor it quickly for an accurate estimate. Multiply the 10-second heart-rate value by six to calculate the heart rate in beats per minute.

Table 10.1 lists THR values for people of different ages with consideration given to present activity status. The THRs are listed as 10-second values because that is the way people commonly refer to THR.

Figure 10.1 demonstrates how to take your pulse at your wrist or neck. One word of caution: If you take it at your neck, don't press too hard because that could result in a slowing of the pulse.

Table 10.1

Estimated 10-Second THR for People Whose HRmax Is Unknown

Population	Intensity % $\dot{V}O_2$max	20	30	40	50	60	70	80
					AGE (YEARS)			
Inactive	50	22	21	20	18	17	16	15
with several	55	23	22	21	19	18	17	16
risk factors	60	24	23	22	20	19	18	17
Normal activity	65	25	24	23	21	20	19	18
with few	70	26	25	24	22	21	20	18
risk factors	75	28	26	25	24	22	21	19
	80	29	28	26	25	23	22	20
Very active	85	30	29	27	26	24	23	21
with low risk	90	31	30	28	27	25	24	22

Reprinted, by permission, from E.T. Howley and B.D. Franks, 1997, *Health Fitness Instructor's Handbook*, 3d ed. (Champaign, IL: Human Kinetics), 277.

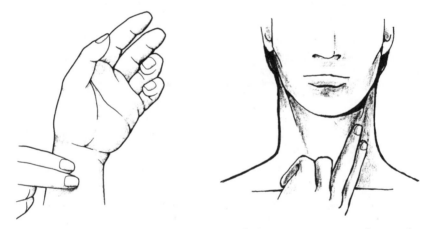

Figure 10.1 Checking your pulse rate: radial—at your wrist, and carotid—at your neck.

Types of Activities

At the beginning of a fitness program we recommend activities that are easily controlled in terms of intensity, provide an adequate means of expending calories, and have a low probability of causing injury. Walking, cycling, and swimming are examples of such activities. Emphasize low intensity and long duration at the start of your program, progressing to more and varied activities as you become more fit.

Orthopedic Problems

If you experience pain in the ankle, knee, or hip when you walk or jog, cut back on the amount of activity that you are doing or change the activity itself (e.g., a jogger can switch to swimming or cycling). If you have a chronic orthopedic problem, choose an activity that will not aggravate it. In addition, you might follow the recommendations in chapter 8 about how to deal with chronic inflammation problems. Generally, it is important to do a long warm-up and use ice afterward to minimize any swelling that may occur. Again, seriously consider an alternative activity that will take a load off the joints that are bothering you. If the condition persists, see your physician.

The direction is from low to high intensity, from more to less controlled, and from activities with a low risk of injury to those representing slightly greater risk.

Maintaining the Recommended Fitness Level

For some people, simply taking long walks may satisfy their needs and accomplish their fitness goals. Others may desire a higher level of fitness so that they can participate in activities such as racquetball, basketball, soccer, tennis, or recreational 10-kilometer (10K) runs. When you have achieved the level you desire, be aware that you must exercise three or four times per week, 30 to 40 minutes per session at your THR to maintain the level. Once you have established a routine of regular exercise, you need to regard your exercise time as one of the most important things in your life, something you schedule other things around. By doing so you will find it easier to maintain your fitness over the years and not experience the "aging effect" to the same extent as the sedentary population.

Where Do I Start and How Do I Progress?

Individuals often ask how to get started in a fitness program and what the next steps are once they get started. The following paragraphs

Guidelines for Exercising With Health Risks

Diabetes

- Work with a physician or nurse educator.
- Adjust medication (if taking any) prior to exercise.
- Increase carbohydrate intake if needed.
- Inform the exercise leader that you are a diabetic.
- Carry along a readily available form of glucose in case of hypoglycemia.
- Exercise with a "buddy" who can help out in an emergency.

Asthma

- Work with your physician to control the asthma with medication.
- Take medication prior to exercise.
- Do a long warm-up and short-interval activities.
- Inform the exercise leader that you have asthma.
- Carry along an aerosol bronchodilator.
- Exercise with a "buddy" who can help out in an emergency.

High Blood Pressure

- Work with your physician to control the hypertension.
- If medication is prescribed, take it regularly.
- Do dynamic endurance activities involving large muscle groups.
- Have your blood pressure measured regularly.

Seizure Disorders

- Take your prescribed medication regularly.
- Inform your exercise leader about your condition.
- Exercise with a "buddy."

Pregnancy

- Work with your physician to plan the exercise program.
- Follow a three-day-per-week pattern, with warm-up and cool-down. Avoid exercising when fatigued and exercising to exhaustion.
- Avoid prolonged activity or activity in hot, humid weather and drink plenty of fluids to maintain hydration.
- Do not perform exercises while lying on your back after the third month of pregnancy.
- Avoid fast (ballistic) movements and deep flexion and extension exercises.

provide recommendations for moving from a sedentary to an active lifestyle. The logical sequence of phases will reduce the chance of injury and improve the potential for lifelong participation.

Phase 1—Daily Activity

The first step is to include more activity as part of your daily routine. Examples include using stairs instead of an escalator or elevator, getting off the bus or train a stop early to walk home or to work, and parking farther from the store to include a short walk when shopping.

Phase 2—Regular Walking

The next step in a fitness program is regular walking. This activity can range from very low to high intensity depending on the speed of the walk, and it can be done in any weather by most people, young or old. We recommend that you be able to walk about four miles at a brisk pace without undue fatigue before moving on to more strenuous activities. A planned program to accomplish that will be presented shortly.

Phase 3—Progress to Recommended Work Levels for Fitness Base

Once you have achieved the goal of the walking program, you may want to begin a walk/jog/run (or swim or bike) program to achieve higher levels of cardiorespiratory fitness. We emphasize the need to progress slowly from one stage of the program to the next in order to minimize muscle soreness and increase the probability of success. The THR zone will act as an intensity guide, helping you select your proper pace and the length of the first stages of the jog/walk program. Aim to be able to jog three miles in the THR zone. A typical walk/jog/run program follows our discussion of the program for walkers.

Phase 4—Fitness Activity Variety

After you have developed a fitness base that allows you to jog three miles comfortably, you are ready to undertake a variety of less controlled fitness games or activities. These often require some skill and have an inherently higher risk of injury. This phase is not for everyone, and it is designed, of course, around your particular interests. We encourage you to develop new skills (an old dog can learn new tricks!) and become involved in a variety of activities. By doing so, you will be at less risk for becoming sedentary. For example, if it is rainy and cold outside, a jogger can substitute racquetball or participate in an aerobic dance class. A runner who hurts a knee can swim or cycle. Games provide a natural framework for establishing a socially supportive environment. Remember, you have to stay active to remain fit.

Samples of Activities

In this section we will provide details of the walking, jogging, cycling, and exercise-to-music (often called "aerobics") programs, as well as comment on some other activities.

Considerations for Walking, Jogging, and Running Programs

When you walk, one foot is always in contact with the ground. When you jog or run, there is a period of "flight" during which both feet are off the ground. The extra energy required to propel the body off the ground and to absorb the force of impact when landing makes jogging or running a better way to expend calories, but the probability of injury is higher as well. It is more difficult to distinguish jogging

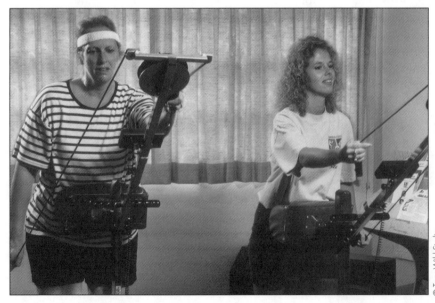

from running. A world-class runner may "jog" through a warm-up at seven miles per hour, while a person of average fitness may be running all out at the same speed. Jogging usually refers to a submaximal running speed.

Shoes

Specialized walking shoes are now available from major shoe manufacturers that are catering to the growing market of walking enthusiasts. For most people, however, a comfortable pair of ordinary shoes offering reasonable side support is sufficient to start a walking program. Specialized walking shoes may be a reasonable investment for someone who has chosen walking as a primary activity. A good-quality pair of jogging/running shoes with the usual cushioning to absorb the shock of impact and the structural support to resist movement of the heels upon landing is also suitable for walking. So, if you are going to be moving from the walking to the jogging/running phases of a fitness program, an investment in a pair of good-quality running shoes is reasonable. We recommend that you buy your shoes at a store that specializes in athletic shoes and that you be fitted late in the day (when your feet are at their largest) wearing the same kind of socks you use during a workout.

Clothing

Choose clothing that makes you feel as comfortable as possible during the exercise session. In hot weather wear loose-fitting, light-colored clothing and a hat with a brim if you are exercising in direct sunlight. Cotton fabrics are recommended—they allow sweat to evaporate. Be careful not to be taken in by advertising that suggests that by wearing plastic, nylon, or rubber clothing you will lose more weight when exercising in warm weather. The weight you lose is water weight, not fat weight, and wearing these fabrics can create a dangerous situation by making it more difficult to keep your body cool.

If you exercise outdoors in the cold weather, wear layers of clothing so that you can remove a layer or two as you warm up and begin to sweat. The idea is not to produce too much sweat, which can accelerate heat loss and may cause a reduction in body temperature. Wool and polypropylene fabrics are recommended because they maintain their insulating qualities even when wet with sweat. A hat and mittens are recommended as you lose a great deal of heat from your head and hands. For those who tend to have cold hands, wearing a pair of polypropylene gloves inside mittens can provide additional comfort. Emphasize comfort, not looks. Based on our observations of the outfits worn by some wintertime joggers, this approach is certainly being followed!

Location and Surface

The first consideration in choosing a workout site is safety. Walking is a good activity; walking in Central Park in New York City after dark is not healthful (or smart!). Consider the traffic flow, lighting, and surface when you select an area. Low-traffic areas are more relaxing and reduce the chance of an accident. If you walk, jog, or run in the streets, be sure to run toward oncoming traffic so you can see what is ahead. In addition, wear bright clothing that is easily visible. Whether you believe you have the right of way or not, yield to traffic at every intersection or commercial driveway.

The surface should be relatively smooth, and you must be aware of cracks, holes, and debris to avoid sprains and strains. The hardness of the surface is not important for those who walk, as the force of impact is relatively low. For those who jog or run, the surface can influence the degree of comfort, especially if you have some arthritis in your ankles, knees, or hips. A soft surface like grass or a cushioned track will relieve some of the problems. When jogging on grass, however, be careful of roots and holes. Given the concern for injuries and safety, the area should be well lighted.

Walking Program

The walking program shown in table 10.2 takes you from a very light level of activity to being able to walk 60 minutes at a brisk pace. We have stated five rules at the top of the table. The most important rule is not to progress to the next stage until you are comfortable at the current stage. Don't be in a rush to get fit. Take your time and enjoy steady progress toward your goal. We recommend that you increase the distance you walk at a slow speed before you increase your speed. We have not stated a particular walking speed because what is comfortable for one person may be too fast or too slow for another.

At the end of the walking program, when you can walk four miles or so at a brisk pace, you are ready to start the jogging program. However, as mentioned earlier, some of you will prefer to stay at the "brisk walk" stage of the walking program as your most intense activity. Walking with a partner or in a group is enjoyable for many fitness participants. The main precaution when exercising together is to take care not to push each other to work beyond what is comfortable.

Table 10.2

Walking Program

Rules:
1. Start at a level that is comfortable to you.
2. Be aware of new aches or pains.
3. Don't progress to next level if not comfortable.
4. Monitor heart rate and record it.
5. It would be healthful to walk at least every other day.

Stage	Duration (min)	Heart rate	Comments
1	15	_____	_____
2	20	_____	_____
3	25	_____	_____
4	30	_____	_____
5	30	_____	_____
6	30	_____	_____
7	35	_____	_____
8	40	_____	_____
9	45	_____	_____
10	45	_____	_____
11	45	_____	_____
12	50	_____	_____
13	55	_____	_____
14	60	_____	_____
15	60	_____	_____
16	60	_____	_____
17	60	_____	_____
18	60	_____	_____
19	60	_____	_____
20	60	_____	_____

Note. From *The Health Fitness Handbook* by B.D. Franks and E.T. Howley, 1999, Champaign, IL: Human Kinetics. This table may be copied by instructors and agencies who have purchased the book.
Reprinted, by permission, from B.D. Franks and E.T. Howley, 1998, *Fitness Leader's Handbook*, 2d ed. (Champaign, IL: Human Kinetics), 124.

Jogging Program

A jogging program is described in table 10.3. The first rule to follow is to complete the walking program. In addition, the first five levels of the program emphasize the need to mix walking with jogging to stay at the low end of the THR zone where you should perceive the exercise as being easy. This gradual transition will result in less muscle soreness. You might consider doing this program on a track, in a park, or on a very quiet street so that you will not have to be concerned with too much traffic or noise. In addition, you might find it more enjoyable if you jog with someone else. The time will fly by and you will have someone to help you along.

In almost every community there are opportunities to compete in running races—one-mile "fun runs" or social 10K (6.2-mile) runs. For people interested in jogging or running as a primary form of activity, these runs can, and should, be fun. The focus of your attention in such runs should be on completing the course comfortably. As you become more fit, you will be able to run the race in a shorter time. Remember, the focus of attention in this book is on becoming fit, not on achieving world-class status as a runner. Those who choose to emphasize competitive running, in which the main goal is to run faster and faster, should expect more injuries and muscle soreness to accompany that endeavor. We advise a similar attitude of focusing on your own progress with walking races.

Cycling Program

A cycling program can use a regular bicycle or one of the many stationary cycle ergometers found in fitness centers. Cycling is a good exercise alternative for people who do not like to jog or run and can also give relief to those who have joint tenderness. Adjust the seat height so that your knee has only a slight bend when your foot is at the bottom of a pedal swing. Table 10.4 outlines a cycling program that progresses in much the same way as the walking and jogging programs. The emphasis at the beginning of the program is on simply riding the equivalent of one or two miles three times a week. After that, work at the low end of the THR zone (around 70 percent of maximal heart rate) until you can comfortably do 15 to 25 minutes of activity. As you progress through the program, stay within your THR zone and do not advance to the next stage until you are comfortable with the present one.

Table 10.3

Jogging Program

Rules:
1. Complete the walking program before starting this program.
2. Begin each session with stretching and walking.
3. Be aware of new aches or pains.
4. Don't progress to next level if not comfortable.
5. Stay at low end of THR zone; record heart rate for each session.
6. Do program on a day-on, day-off basis.

Stage 1 Jog 10 steps, walk 10 steps. Repeat five times and take your heart rate. Stay within THR zone by increasing or decreasing walking phase. Do 20 to 30 min of activity.

Stage 2 Jog 20 steps, walk 10 steps. Repeat five times and take your heart rate. Stay within THR zone by increasing or decreasing walking phase. Do 20 to 30 min of activity.

Stage 3 Jog 30 steps, walk 10 steps. Repeat five times and take your heart rate. Stay within THR zone by increasing or decreasing walking phase. Do 20 to 30 min of activity.

Stage 4 Jog 1 min, walk 10 steps. Repeat three times and take your heart rate. Stay within THR zone by increasing or decreasing walking phase. Do 20 to 30 min of activity.

Stage 5 Jog 2 min, walk 10 steps. Repeat two times and take your heart rate. Stay within THR zone by increasing or decreasing walking phase. Do 30 min of activity.

Stage 6 Jog 1 lap (400 m, or 440 yd) and check heart rate. Adjust pace during run to stay within the THR zone. If heart rate is still too high, go back to the Stage 5 schedule. Do 6 laps with a brief walk between each.

Stage 7 Jog 2 laps and check heart rate. Adjust pace during run to stay within the THR zone. If heart rate is still too high, go back to the Stage 6 activity. Do 6 laps with a brief walk between each.

Stage 8 Jog 1 mi and check heart rate. Adjust pace during the run to stay within the THR zone. Do 2 mi.

Stage 9 Jog 2–3 mi continuously. Check heart rate at the end to ensure that you were within THR zone.

Note. From *The Health Fitness Handbook* by B.D. Franks and E.T. Howley, 1999, Champaign, IL: Human Kinetics. This table may be copied by instructors and agencies who have purchased the book.
Reprinted, by permission, from B.D. Franks and E.T. Howley, 1998, *Fitness Leader's Handbook*, 2d ed. (Champaign, IL: Human Kinetics), 125.

Table 10.4

Cycling Program

Rules:
1. Start at a level that is comfortable for you.
2. Use either a regular bicycle or a stationary exercise cycle.
3. If you are starting at stage 1, simply get used to riding 1 or 2 miles. Don't be concerned about time or reaching the lower end of your target heart rate (THR) zone.

Stage	Distance (mi)	THR (% of max HR)	Time (min)	Frequency (days/week)
1	1–2	—	—	3
2	1–2	60	8–12	3
3	3–5	60	15–25	3
4	6–8	70	25–35	3
5	6–8	70	25–35	4
6	10–15	70	40–60	4
7	10–15	80	35–50	4–5

Note. From *The Health Fitness Handbook* by B.D. Franks and E.T. Howley, 1999, Champaign, IL: Human Kinetics. This table may be copied by instructors and agencies who have purchased the book.
Reprinted, by permission, from B.D. Franks and E.T. Howley, 1998, *Fitness Leader's Handbook*, 2d ed. (Champaign, IL: Human Kinetics), 126.

Games and Sports

Games and some sports can be used in a fitness program, and for the reasons already mentioned, we encourage interested individuals to do so. However, we also recommend that a person first be able to move through the walking and the jogging programs. These programs emphasize more controlled types of activity at an intensity that will help you achieve cardiovascular fitness levels and change body composition to facilitate your involvement in a game. If you are not fit enough to play a game, then the possibility of having fun is diminished and the possibility of injury is increased.

Games can help you achieve fitness if they are vigorous (i.e., you reach your THR zone) and are somewhat sustained so that you are exercising at your THR for 30 to 40 minutes. If you stand around or are excluded (e.g., sitting on the bench), games are not very useful in expending energy or raising morale. Many games require skill in order to participate in a meaningful way, and when one or both parties in a doubles game lack that skill, neither gets a workout. It is important that the participants are well matched in terms of skill level. If a skill difference exists between players in a sport such as racquetball or tennis, there is a good chance that both will spend more time in flexibility exercises (picking up the ball) than in exercise that improves cardiorespiratory function. To make the transition from jogging to a particular game, you might continue your normal workouts and learn the game gradually.

Exercise leaders in some fitness programs use low-organized games as fitness activities. These activities require minimal skill, and the fun level is maximal. The games can be controlled easily to keep all participants in their respective THR zones. In such games, you need to judge when the game is becoming too much for you. The goal is to have fun and be fit, and games can certainly meet those requirements.

Aquatic Activities

Swimming is an excellent alternative to playing games, running, or cycling to achieve a cardiorespiratory training effect. Aquatic activities, however, include more than just swimming. You can walk, jog, or run in the water; hold onto the side of the pool and do flexibility exercises; or play games in the water. Swimming or one of these other activities is a good choice if you have a chronic orthopedic problem or a recent injury that will not allow you to do your regular workout. Water supports your weight to relieve the load on ankles, knees, and hips while providing enough resistance to expend a large number of calories and achieve THR.

Target Heart Rate in Water

Your maximal heart rate is about 13 beats per minute lower when you are immersed in water. This shifts the THR zone back about 10 beats per minute, since it is dependent on your maximal heart rate. When you exercise in water, therefore, you do not have to achieve the same THR value as you do on land to reach the exercise intensity that results in a training effect.

Progression

Progress from low-intensity to higher-intensity activities in the pool in much the same way that you do on land. You can do flexibility activities by moving your legs forward, backward, and to the side in a gentle and easy motion while holding onto the side of the pool with one hand. You can also hang onto the side of the pool with both hands so that your body is floating and practice some of the kicking that is part of regular swimming. Those who cannot swim can walk or jog across the pool while doing a swimming stroke. Water offers enough resistance to this movement so that most people can achieve their THR. You can vary this by walking backward or skipping side to side while moving across the pool. Flotation devices can also offer a good deal of resistance while providing support. In this way, even a nonswimmer can achieve a satisfying workout while "swimming" up and down the pool.

Swimming laps in the pool requires a certain level of skill. A poor swimmer will be exhausted at the end of one or two laps and will be unable to complete the workout needed to expend the necessary 200 to 300 calories. If you are a nonswimmer or a poor swimmer, however, take heart. Learning to swim or improving your stroke can happen at any age. In addition to its survival value, swimming provides an alternative when other exercise activities cannot be done due to injury, disease (such as arthritis), or situation.

Learn the simplest strokes first and gradually work up to others. Check your heart rate during the swimming workout as you would for running. The distance one must swim to expend 300 or so calories varies with the stroke used and the swimmer's skill level (see table 5.10). A very rough rule of thumb is that a one-mile swim is equal to about four miles of jogging. Begin each workout with a gradual warm-up and finish with a cool-down.

Table 10.5 outlines the stages of a swimming program. You can start your swimming program at any of the stages, depending on your skill and current fitness levels. Also, don't hesitate to vary the components to suit your needs. For example, you might like to jog four widths, swim four widths, and walk two widths, repeating the sequence to achieve 20 to 30 minutes of activity at your THR. Simply remember to take your time in making the transition to longer duration and more intense activities.

Exercising to Music

One of the best things to happen to fitness exercises in the past 30 years was setting them to music. It has provided an exercise opportunity for people who do not like to jog or run. In addition, exercising to music provides one less excuse to those of us who would skip our exercise sessions because the weather is (pick one) too hot, too cold, too wet, and so on.

Table 10.5

Swimming Program

Rules:
1. Start at a level that is comfortable to you.
2. Don't progress to next stage if not comfortable with current one.
3. Monitor and record heart rate.

Stage 1 In chest-deep water, walk across the width of the pool four times and see if you are close to THR. Gradually increase the duration of the walk until you can do two 10-min walks at THR.

Stage 2 In chest-deep water, walk across and jog back. Repeat twice and see if you are close to THR. Gradually increase the duration of the jogging until you can complete four 5-min jogs at THR.

Stage 3 In chest-deep water, walk across and swim back (any stroke). Use kickboard or flotation device if needed. Repeat this cycle twice and see if you are at THR. Keep up this pattern of walk–swim to do about 20 to 30 min of activity.

Stage 4 In chest-deep water, jog across and swim back (any stroke); repeat and check THR. Gradually decrease the duration of the jog and increase the duration of the swim until four widths can be completed within the THR zone. Accomplish 20 to 30 min of activity per session.

Stage 5 Slowly swim 25 yards, rest 30 seconds, slowly swim another 25 yards, and check THR. On the basis of the heart-rate response, change the speed of the swim and/or the length of the rest period to stay within the THR zone. Gradually increase the number of lengths you can swim (three, then four, and so on) before checking THR.

Stage 6 Increase the duration of continuous swimming until you can accomplish 20 to 30 min without a rest.

Note. From *The Health Fitness Handbook* by B.D. Franks and E.T. Howley, 1999, Champaign, IL: Human Kinetics. This table may be copied by instructors and agencies who have purchased the book.
Reprinted, by permission, from B.D. Franks and E.T. Howley, 1998, *Fitness Leader's Handbook*, 2d ed. (Champaign, IL: Human Kinetics), 129.

Advantages

Music provides a sense of pace and the camaraderie to keep at it, in contrast to other, more isolated activities such as cycling, jogging on a treadmill, or swimming laps in a pool. The pace can be varied by the tempo of the music, which becomes a distraction from the exercise as you listen to the changing rhythms. In addition, musical exercise sessions offer a better balance of activities to achieve fitness goals in flexibility, muscular endurance, and cardiorespiratory endurance. Generally speaking, you will have no problem reaching your THR during a session. In fact, you may find it easy to reach your THR, and we recommend that you do too little rather than too much as you begin this type of exercise. Emphasize enjoying the session, not competing with others, either in the types of steps you use or in continuing when your body is telling you to slow down. As we mentioned earlier, the idea of "no pain, no gain," still heard in some health clubs, is wrong! "Train, don't strain" is more appropriate and will bring you more benefits in the long run.

Disadvantages

The reason for doing too little rather than too much is that exercise-to-music programs lead to their share of injuries. The routines tend to isolate smaller muscle groups and skeletal structures. In addition, people may start this kind of activity program before they are ready. We recommend that you achieve a minimum level of fitness (an ability to complete a four-mile walk) before undertaking this kind of activity. Further, we suggest that you vary this kind of exercise with others that do not put as much stress on joints, such as cycling and swimming.

Level

Fitness centers now offer a wider variety of exercise-to-music classes than they did in the past. This is due partly to the incidence of injuries in regular-level classes and partly to the recognized need to offer classes suited to older and more sedentary individuals. It is reasonable to start with beginner and low-impact classes and move up to more advanced classes as your fitness and interest grow.

Choosing a Good Fitness Program

Choose a fitness program based on your current interests, goals, and ability to follow through on the program. If you choose a program that is difficult to get to or meets at times that conflict with home or work commitments, then you are getting into a situation that may be self-defeating. We recommend that you begin with a basic walking program that will prepare you for more strenuous exercise and help you structure your schedule to start a more formal program, if that is your choice. As you are working on this, you might investigate the fitness clubs in your area. Find out what kinds of programs are of-

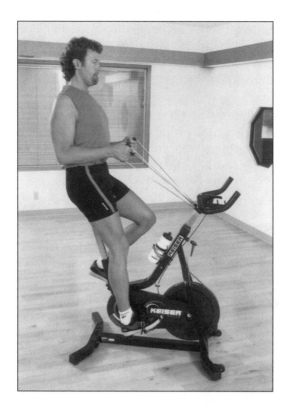

fered and the qualifications of the employees. Good programs hire fitness instructors who have been certified by an outside agency such as the American College of Sports Medicine. A good fitness program offers dynamic exercises done three or four times per week at an intensity that allows you to exercise long enough to expend 200 to 300 calories. The number of calories used in common fitness activities is presented in chapter 5.

Beyond Exercise

This book presents the information necessary to begin and continue a safe and healthy exercise program. We have assumed that you are interested in fitness in order to improve your health. In this final section of the chapter we discuss the direct and indirect values of exercise. These are our subjective observations and we hope they will stimulate you to consider the ways in which exercise is meaningful to you.

Physical activity can be valuable in our lives in and of itself, even if it had no physical health benefits. Depending on the activity and the environment in which it is done, exercise can meet some of our seemingly opposite needs. It can help us whether we need to be

- learning discipline or having fun,
- serious or frivolous,
- alone with our thoughts or enjoying others, or
- using time wisely or not using time badly.

When we exercise regularly, we may feel good just knowing we have the discipline to complete a workout even on busy days. At other times, the workout is fun for its own sake as we move our bodies in different ways, play games with modified rules, or simply become aware of our natural surroundings while exercising. Exercise can allow for serious contemplation of an upcoming task or a replay of a major life event. At other times, exercise is done in the most frivolous way as we joke with our exercise companions. Because of the benefits of exercise, we are using our time wisely. At the same time, exercise uses time that we might otherwise have used in unhealthy ways (e.g., eating junk food, smoking, or watching TV).

If you feel you are not reaping some of the rewards of exercise, try other forms or environments. For example, if you normally exercise with others, try taking a long walk or jog by yourself before an important speech or decision.

Another important aspect of physical activity is the freedom it affords us. Increased health and vitality enhance our lives at home, at work, and in our leisure and help us approach these other parts of our lives with a positive attitude. If you don't experience these results from your exercise program, consider making some modifications.

One major factor determines whether physical activity will bring you its full benefits: *you*. Are you willing to exercise even when your life is hectic, the weather is lousy, and no one calls you to play? Will you give regular exercise the same priority status as eating, sleeping, and brushing your teeth? Your health and physical well-being are worth a few hours a week. Decide that you are going to begin a fitness program and continue it for the rest of your life *starting now*.

Health Status Questionnaire

Table A.1

Health Status Questionnaire

Instructions

Complete each question accurately. All information provided is confidential if you choose to submit this form to your fitness instructor.

Part 1. Information about the individual

1. _____   _____
   Legal name   Nickname

2. _____   _____
   Mailing address   Home phone

   _____   _____
                                               Business phone

3. *EI* _____   _____
   Personal physician   Phone

   _____
   Address

4. *EI* _____   _____
   Person to contact in emergency   Phone

5. Gender (circle one):   Female   Male *(RF)*

6. *RF* Date of birth: _____
                        Month   Day   Year

7. Number of hours worked per week (circle one):   < 20   20–40   41–60   > 60

8. *SLA* More than 25% of time spent on job (circle all that apply)
       Sitting at desk   Lifting or carrying loads   Standing   Walking   Driving

9. Briefly describe your occupation, including part-time jobs: _____

   _____

   _____

Part 2. Medical history

10. *RF* Family medical history (List only immediate family members such as grandparents, mother, father, siblings, children.)

Alcoholism/drug abuse *SEP*	Emphysema *SEP*	Infectious mononucleosis *MC*
Allergies	Epilepsy *SEP*	Kidney problem *MC*
Anemia *SEP*	Eye problems *SLA*	Mental illness *SEP*
Asthma *SEP*	Head trauma *MC*	Neck strain *SLA*
Back strain *SLA*	Hearing loss *SLA*	Obesity *RF*
Bleeding trait *SEP*	Heart problem *MC*	Phlebitis *MC*
Bronchitis, chronic *SEP*	Hepatitis	Rheumatoid arthritis *SLA*
Cancer *SEP*	Hernia	Sickle cell disease or trait *SEP*
Cirrhosis, liver *MC*	High blood pressure *RF*	Stroke *MC*
Congenital defect *SEP*	Hypoglycemia *SEP*	Thyroid problem *SEP*
Diabetes *SEP*	Hyperlipidemia *RF*	Ulcer *SEP*
		Other _____

Please note any other diseases that run in your family that you are aware of:

_____

Please indicate any family members who have or have had the following before age 55:

Heart attack _____ Stroke _____ High blood pressure _____

If any family member has died, please list age and cause of death (write "unknown" if applicable):

Family member	Age at death	Cause of death
_____	_____	_____
_____	_____	_____
_____	_____	_____

Current age of parents if they are living: Mother _____ Father _____

11. Date of

Last medical physical exam: _____ (Year)

Last physical fitness test: _____ (Year)

12. Were you ever hospitalized or have you had any outpatient surgery? If yes, please write date and describe.

_____

_____

_____

13. Please circle any of the following for which you have been diagnosed or treated by a physician or health professional:

Alcoholism/Drug abuse *SEP*	Epilepsy *SEP*	Kidney problem *MC*
Allergies	Eye problems *SLA*	Mental illness *SEP*
Anemia *SEP*	Head trauma *MC*	Neck strain *SLA*
Asthma *SEP*	Hearing loss *SLA*	Obesity *RF*
Back strain *SLA*	Heart problem *MC*	Phlebitis *MC*
Bleeding trait *SEP*	Hepatitis	Rheumatoid arthritis *SLA*
Bronchitis, chronic *SEP*	Hernia	Sickle cell disease or trait *SEP*
Cancer *SEP*	High blood pressure *RF*	Stroke *MC*
Cirrhosis, liver *MC*	Hypoglycemia *SEP*	Thyroid problem *SEP*
Congenital defect *SEP*	Hyperlipidemia *RF*	Ulcer *SEP*
Diabetes *SEP*	Infectious mononucleosis *MC*	Other _____
Emphysema *SEP*		

14. Circle all medicine taken in last 6 months:

Blood thinner *MC*	Heart rhythm medication *MC*	Pain medication
Bronchodilators	High blood pressure	Seizure medication *SEP*
Medicine for diabetes *SEP*	medication *MC*	Steroids
Digitalis *MC*	Insulin *MC*	Other _____
Diuretic *MC*	Nitroglycerin *MC*	

15. Frequent occurence of any of the following symptoms may indicate the need for medical attention. Circle the number indicating how often you have experienced each of the following:

> 5 = Very often
> 4 = Fairly often
> 3 = Sometimes
> 2 = Infrequently
> 1 = Practically never

Chronic cough *MC*	1	2	3	4	5
Abdominal pain *MC*	1	2	3	4	5
Low back pain *MC*	1	2	3	4	5
Joint/extremity pain *MC*	1	2	3	4	5
Chest pain *RF MC*	1	2	3	4	5
Feeling faint *MC*	1	2	3	4	5
Dizziness *MC*	1	2	3	4	5
Shortness of breath with slight exertion	1	2	3	4	5
Lumps	1	2	3	4	5
Hoarseness	1	2	3	4	5
Varicose veins	1	2	3	4	5
Numbness of extremities	1	2	3	4	5
Constipation or diarrhea	1	2	3	4	5
Memory loss	1	2	3	4	5
Confusion or coordination difficulty	1	2	3	4	5
Sleep problems	1	2	3	4	5
Palpitation or fast heart beat	1	2	3	4	5
Unusual fatigue with normal activity *MC*	1	2	3	4	5
Skin color change	1	2	3	4	5
Trouble controlling anger	1	2	3	4	5
Urination problems	1	2	3	4	5
Loss of sense of smell or taste	1	2	3	4	5

Part 3. Health-related behavior

16. *RF* Do you currently smoke?   Yes   No

17. *RF* If you are a smoker, indicate number smoked per day:

Cigarettes: 40 or more   20–39   10–19   1–9

Cigars or pipes only: 5 or more, or any inhaled   Less than 5, none inhaled

18. *RF* Do you exercise regularly?   Yes   No

19. How many days per week do you accumulate 30 minutes of moderate activity?

> 0   1   2   3   4   5   6   7

20. How many days per week do you normally spend at least 20 minutes in vigorous exercise?

    0   1   2   3   4   5   6   7

21. Can you walk 4 miles briskly without fatigue?   Yes   No

22. Can you jog 3 miles continuously at a moderate pace without discomfort?   Yes   No

23. Weight now: _____ lb   One year ago: _____ lb   At age 21: _____ lb

Part 4. Health-related attitudes

24. *RF* Certain traits have been associated with coronary-prone behavior. Circle the number that corresponds to your degree of agreement or disagreement with the following statements:

    6 = Strongly agree   3 = Slightly disagree
    5 = Moderately agree   2 = Moderately disagree
    4 = Slightly agree   1 = Strongly disagree

    I am an impatient, time-conscious, hard-driving individual.

    1   2   3   4   5   6

25. List everything not already included on this questionnaire that might cause you problems in a fitness test or fitness program.

    _____

    _____

    _____

Code for Health Status Questionnaire

The following code will help you evaluate the information in the Health Status Questionnaire.

EI = Emergency Information—must be readily available.

MC = Medical Clearance needed—do not participate in exercise without physician's permission.

SEP = Special Emergency Procedures needed—do not exercise alone; make sure your exercise partner knows what to do in case of an emergency.

RF = Risk Factor for CHD—educational materials and workshops needed.

SLA = Special or Limited Activities may be needed—you may need to include or exclude specific exercises.

OTHER (not marked) = Personal information that may be helpful for files or research.

Adapted, by permission, from E.T. Howley and B.D. Franks, 1997, *Health Fitness Instructor's Handbook,* 3d ed. (Champaign, IL: Human Kinetics), 34–36.

Recommended Dietary Allowances and Intakes

Table B.1

Recommended Daily Dietary Allowances for Adults

Age (years) or Condition	Weight (kg)	Weight (lb)	Height (cm)	Height (in.)	Protein (g)	FAT-SOLUBLE VITAMINS Vita- min A (μg RE)	Vita- min D (mg)	Vita- min E (mg α-TE)	Vita- min K (mg)
Males									
15–18	66	145	176	69	59	1,000	10	10	65
19–24	72	160	177	70	58	1,000	10	10	70
25–50	79	174	176	70	63	1,000	5	10	80
51+	77	170	173	68	63	1,000	5	10	80
Females									
15–18	55	120	163	64	44	800	10	8	55
19–24	58	128	164	65	46	800	10	8	60
25–50	63	138	163	64	50	800	5	8	65
51+	65	143	160	63	50	800	5	8	65
Pregnant					60	800	10	10	65
Lactating									
First 6 months					65	1,300	10	12	65
Second 6 months					62	1,200	10	11	65

(continued)

Table B.1 *(continued)*

WATER-SOLUBLE VITAMINS

Age (years) or Condition	Vita-min C (mg)	Thia-min (mg)	Ribo-flavin (mg)	Niacin (mg NE)	Vita-min B$_6$ (mg)	Folate (μg)	Vita-min B$_{12}$ (μg)
Males							
15–18	60	1.5	1.8	20	2.0	200	2.0
19–24	60	1.5	1.7	19	2.0	200	2.0
25–50	60	1.5	1.7	19	2.0	200	2.0
51+	60	1.2	1.4	15	2.0	200	2.0
Females							
15–18	60	1.1	1.3	15	1.5	180	2.0
19–24	60	1.1	1.3	15	1.6	180	2.0
25–50	60	1.1	1.3	15	1.6	180	2.0
51+	60	1.0	1.2	13	1.6	180	2.0
Pregnant	70	1.5	1.6	17	2.2	400	2.2
Lactating							
First 6 months	95	1.6	1.8	20	2.1	280	2.6
Second 6 months	90	1.6	1.7	20	2.1	260	2.6

MINERALS

Age (years) or Condition	Cal-cium (mg)	Phos-phorus (mg)	Mag-nesium (mg)	Iron (mg)	Zinc (mg)	Iodine (μg)	Sele-nium (μg)
Males							
15–18	1,200	1,200	400	12	15	150	50
19–24	1,200	1,200	350	10	15	150	70
25–50	800	800	350	10	15	150	70
51+	800	800	350	10	15	150	70
Females							
15–18	1,200	1,200	300	15	12	150	50
19–24	1,200	1,200	280	15	12	150	55
25–50	800	800	280	15	12	150	55
51+	800	800	280	10	12	150	55
Pregnant	1,200	1,200	320	30	15	175	65
Lactating							
First 6 months	1,200	1,200	355	15	19	200	75
Second 6 months	1,200	1,200	340	15	16	200	75

National Research Council. *Recommended Dietary Allowances*, 10th ed. National Academy of Sciences, 1989.

Table B.2

Recommended Dietary Reference Intakes

Life-stage/ Group	Calcium (mg/d)	Phosphorus (mg/d)	Magnesium (mg/d)	D (mg/d)[1,2]	Fluoride (mg/d)	Thiamin (mg/d)
Males						
14–18 y	1,300	**1,250**	410	5	3	**1.2**
19–30 y	1,000	**700**	400	5	4	**1.2**
31–50 y	1,000	**700**	420	5	4	**1.2**
51–70 y	1,200	**700**	420	10	4	**1.2**
> 70 y	1,200	**700**	420	15	4	**1.2**
Females						
14–18 y	1,300	**1,250**	360	5	3	**1.0**
19–30 y	1,000	**700**	310	5	3	**1.1**
31–50 y	1,000	**700**	320	5	3	**1.1**
51–70 y	1,200	**700**	320	10	3	**1.1**
> 70 y	1,200	**700**	320	15	3	**1.1**
Pregnant women						
< 18 y	1,300	**1,250**	400	5	3	**1.4**
19–30 y	1,000	**700**	350	5	3	**1.4**
31–50 y	1,000	**700**	360	5	3	**1.4**
Lactating women						
< 18 y	1,300	**1,250**	360	5	3	**1.5**
19–30 y	1,000	**700**	310	5	3	**1.5**
31–50 y	1,000	**700**	320	5	3	**1.5**

(continued)

Recommended Dietary Allowances (RDAs) appear in bold type and Adequate Intakes (AIs) in ordinary type.

[1] As cholecalciferol: 1 μg of cholecalciferol = 40 IU of vitamin D.

[2] In the absence of adequate exposure to sunlight.

[3] As niacin equivalents: 1 mg of niacin = 60 mg of tryptophan.

[4] As dietary folate equivalents (DFE): 1 DFE = 1 μg of food folate = 0.6 μg of folic acid (from fortified food or supplement) consumed with food = 0.5 μg of synthetic (supplemental) folic acid taken on an empty stomach.

[5] Although AIs have been set for choline, there are few data to assess whether a dietary supply of choline is always needed; it is possible that the choline requirement can be met by endogenous synthesis at certain times.

Table B.2 (continued)

Life-stage/ Group	Ribo-flavin (mg/d)	Niacin (mg/d)[3]	B_6 (mg/d)	Folate (μg/d)[4]	B_{12} (μg/d)	Panto-thenic acid (mg/d)	Biotin (μg/d)	Choline (mg/d)[5]
Males								
14–18 y	1.3	16	1.3	400	2.4	5	25	550
19–30 y	1.3	16	1.3	400	2.4	5	30	550
31–50 y	1.3	16	1.3	400	2.4	5	30	550
51–70 y	1.3	16	1.7	400	2.4#	5	30	550
> 70 y	1.3	16	1.7	400	2.4#	5	30	550
Females								
14–18 y	1.0	14	1.2	400*	2.4	5	25	400
19–30 y	1.1	14	1.3	400*	2.4	5	30	425
31–50 y	1.1	14	1.3	400*	2.4	5	30	425
51–70 y	1.1	14	1.5	400*	2.4#	5	30	425
> 70 y	1.1	14	1.5	400	2.4#	5	30	425
Pregnant women								
< 18 y	1.4	18	1.9	600**	2.6	6	30	450
19–30 y	1.4	18	1.9	600**	2.6	6	30	450
31–50 y	1.4	18	1.9	600**	2.6	6	30	450
Lactating women								
< 18 y	1.6	17	2.0	500	2.8	7	35	550
19–30 y	1.6	17	2.0	500	2.8	7	35	550
31–50 y	1.6	17	2.0	500	2.8	7	35	550

#Since 10% to 30% of older people may malabsorb food-bound B_{12}, those older than 50 years need to meet their RDA mainly by taking foods fortified with B_{12} or a B_{12}-containing supplement.

*In view of evidence linking folate intake with neural tube defects in the fetus, women capable of becoming pregnant need to consume 400 μg of synthetic folic acid from fortified foods and/or supplements in addition to intake of food folate from a varied diet.

**It is assumed that women will continue taking 400 μg of folic acid until their pregnancy is confirmed and they enter prenatal care, which ordinarily occurs after the end of the periconceptional period—the critical time for formation of the neural tube.

Adapted from Food and Nutrition Board, Committee on the Scientific Evaluation of Dietary Reference Intakes. *Dietary Reference Intakes for Calcium, Phosphorus, Magnesium, Vitamin D, and Fluoride.* 1998[1]; Food and Nutrition Board, Committee on the Scientific Evaluation of Dietary Reference Intakes. *Dietary Reference Intakes for Thiamin, Riboflavin, Niacin, Vitamin B$_6$, Folate, Vitamin B$_{12}$, Pantothenic Acid, Biotin, and Choline.* 1998.[2]

Bibliography

The information in *The Health Fitness Handbook* is based on the latest research and official position stands by respected organizations, as summarized in the following references. In order to make the book "user-friendly" and easy to read, we have not documented the sources for individual elements of the book. Those interested in more precise documentation should refer to Howley and Franks (1997).

American College of Obstetricians and Gynecologists. (1985). *Exercise during pregnancy and the postnatal period* (ACOG Home Exercise Program). Washington, DC: Author.

American College of Sports Medicine. (1983). Proper and improper weight loss programs. *Medicine and Science in Sports and Exercise, 15,* ix–xiii.

American College of Sports Medicine. (1995). *Guidelines for exercise testing and prescription* (5th ed.). Philadelphia: Williams & Wilkins.

American Diabetes Association. (1990). Diabetes and exercise: Position statement. *Diabetes Care, 13,* 804–805.

American Diabetes Association and American Dietetic Association. (1986). *Exchange lists* (p. 5). Alexandria, VA and Chicago, IL: Author.

American Heart Association. (1992). Exercise standards: A statement for health care professionals from the American Heart Association. *Circulation, 86,* 340–344.

Blair, S.N., Painter, P., Pate, R.R., Smith, L.K., and Taylor, C.B. (Eds.). (1988). *Resource manual for exercise testing and prescription.* Philadelphia: Lea & Febiger.

Bouchard, C., Shephard, R.J., and Stephens, T. (Eds.). (1994). *Physical activity, fitness, and health.* Champaign, IL: Human Kinetics.

Franks, B.D., and Howley, E.T. (1998). *Fitness leader's handbook* (2nd ed.). Champaign, IL: Human Kinetics.

Golding, L.A., Myers, C.R., and Sinning, W.E. (1989). *The Y's way to physical fitness.* Champaign, IL: Human Kinetics.

Howley, E.T., and Franks, B.D. (1997). *Health fitness instructor's handbook* (3rd ed.). Champaign, IL: Human Kinetics.

Jackson, A.S., and Pollock, M.L. (1985). Practical assessment of body composition. *The Physician and Sportsmedicine, 13,* 76–90.

Johns, R.E., Bloswick, D.S., Elegante, J.M., and Colledge, A.L. (1994). Chronic, recurrent low back pain. *Journal of Occupational Medicine, 36,* 537–547.

Kline, G.M., Porcari, J.P., Hintermeister, R., Freedson, P.S., Ward, A., McCarron, R.F., Ross, J., and Rippe, J.M. (1987). Estimation of $\dot{V}O_2$max from a one-mile track walk, gender, age, and body weight. *Medicine and Science in Sports and Exercise, 19,* 253–259.

Lohman, T.G. (1987). The use of skinfolds to estimate body fatness in children and youth. *Journal of Physical Education, Recreation and Dance, 58*(9), 98–102.

McKenzie, R. (1993). *Treat your own back.* Waikanae, New Zealand: Spinal Publications, Ltd.

Montoye, H.J., Kemper, H.C.G., Saris, W.H.M., and Washburn, R.A. (1996). *Measuring physical activity and energy expenditure.* Champaign, IL: Human Kinetics.

Morrow, J.R., and Gill, D.L. (Eds.). (1995). The Academy Papers: The role of physical activity in fitness and health. *Quest, 47*(3), 1–140.

National Heart, Lung, and Blood Institute, National Institutes of Health. (1996). *NIH consensus development conference on physical activity and cardiovascular health.* Washington, DC: Author.

National Institute of Occupational Safety and Health. (1997). Work practices guide for manual lifting, U.S. Public Health Service. Publication No. 81–122. Akron, OH: American Industrial Hygiene Association.

National Research Council, Food and Nutrition Board. (1989). *Recommended dietary allowances* (10th ed.). Washington, DC: National Academy Press.

Nieman, D.C. (1995). *Fitness and sports medicine: A health-related approach* (3rd ed.). Loma Linda, CA: Bull.

Pate, R.R., Pratt, M., Blair, S.N., Haskell, W.L., Marcera, C.A., and Bouchard, C. (1995). Physical activity and public health: A recommendation from the Centers for Disease Control and Prevention and the American College of Sports Medicine. *Journal of the American Medical Association, 273*(5), 402–407.

Pollock, M.L., and Wilmore, J.H. (1990). *Exercise in health and disease* (2nd ed.). Philadelphia: Saunders.

Powers, S.K., and Howley, E.T. (1997). *Exercise physiology* (3rd ed.). Dubuque, IA: Brown & Benchmark.

U.S. Department of Agriculture and U.S. Department of Health and Human Services. (1996). *Dietary guidelines for Americans* (4th ed.). Washington, DC: Author.

U.S. Department of Health and Human Services. (1991). *Healthy people 2000: National health promotion and disease prevention objectives.* DHHS publication PHS 91-50212. Washington, DC: Author.

U.S. Department of Health and Human Services. (1996). *Surgeon General's Report on physical activity and health.* Washington, DC: Author.

Index

About the Authors

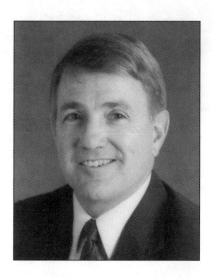

B. Don Franks is a professor in and chair of the Department of Kinesiology at the University of Maryland. Franks is a Fellow of the American College of Sports Medicine (ACSM), the American Academy of Kinesiology and Physical Education (AAKPE), and the Research Consortium of the American Alliance for Health, Physical Education, Recreation and Dance (AAHPERD). He is also a former president of AAKPE and the Research Consortium of AAHPERD. He was Senior Program Advisor for the President's Council on Physical Fitness and Sports in 1995, and he received that group's Distinguished Service Award the following year. He received his PhD in exercise science from the University of Illinois at Urbana-Champaign. Franks lives in Silver Spring, MD.